Body Fix, Body Fit

Body Fix, Body Fit

60 Daily Habits to Keep You on the Move

TRISH FORMBY

ILLUSTRATIONS BY MUDD BEXLEY

Publisher: Badger Books Ltd, 2024

All rights reserved. No part of this publication may be reproduced, distributed, or transmitted in any form or by any means, including photocopying, recording, or other electronic or mechanical methods, without the prior written permission of the copyright holder and the publisher, except in the case of brief quotations embodied in critical reviews and certain other non-commercial uses permitted by copyright law.

The moral right of Trish Formby to be identified as the author and compiler of this work has been asserted.

© Trish Formby, 2025

Second Edition

978-1-0685854-4-9 – Print
978-1-0685854-5-6 – eBook

Insta: @izustrations

Cover and interior illustrations by Mudd Bexley.

Book design by Principal Publishing.

Publisher website: nialledworthy.com

Email: niall@nialledworthy.com

Insta: @nialledworthybooks

For Matt, Jack, Luke and Banjo

Contents

Foreword xi
Hit the Reset Button (Relaxation) 1
Hit the Floor (Pelvis, Core) 3
A Leg To Stand On (Balance) 5
Skating on Thin Ice (Glutes) 7
Bow & Arrow (Upper Back) 9
Backtrack (Legs, Brain!) 11
All Rise (Calves) 13
Super Pooper Trooper (Bowels) 15
Get off Your Butt! (Glutes) 17
Don't get the Hump (Upper Back) 19
Ministry of Funny Walks (Lower Body, Core) 21
Pillow Talk (Sleep Comfort) 23
Rear like a Cobra (Back Extension) 25
Walk like an Egyptian (Shoulders) 27
Bridge the Gap (Thighs, Bums and Tums) 29
Wood Chop (Whole Body, Functional) 31
Core Blimey (Core) 33
Don't Wait for an Emergency to Take the Stairs
 (Whole Body) 35
The Gardener's Joy… and Pain (Lower Back, Knees) .. 37
DIY stands for Don't Injure Yourself (Whole Body) ... 39
Throw the Towel In (Back, Neck, Breathing) 41
Chin Up, Old Boy (Neck, Shoulders) 43
Roll Up! Roll Up! (Back) 45

Make That Trunk Call (Back, Arms) 47
Go on, Give Us a Smile (Happiness!) 49
Bent Knee Calf Raise (Calf) 51
Kitchen Disco (Cardio) 53
Muscling In (Arms) 55
Side Hustle (Back) 57
The Thin End of the Wedge (Back, Thighs) 59
Twist in the Tail (Trunk Rotation) 61
Walk the Plank (Core, Shoulders) 63
Would You Like Ice with That? (Injury) 65
Feel The Heat (Injury) 67
Ski Lifts & Ski Slopes (General) 69
Sitting Pretty (Sitting Posture) 71
Horsing Around (Hamstrings) 73
We Have Lift-Off (Shoulders, Arms) 75
You're a Pushover (Shoulders, Arms) 77
Hip & Bendy (Hip) 79
Child's Play (Whole Body) 81
Get a Grip (Hand, Wrist) 83
Where's Your Head At? (Neck) 85
Housework (Whole Body – and some) 87
Pass the Baton (Forearms, Elbows) 89
The Ankle Angle (Ankle & More!) 91
Stand like a Stork (Legs) 93
Side Plank (Shoulders, Glutes) 95
Prepare for Landing! (Balance) 97
Walk and Talk (Whole Body) 99
Backpacking (Back) 101

Hovercraft (Whole Body) *103*
Do the Pike (Legs, Shoulders) *105*
Salute Your Unsung Little Heroes (Adductors) *107*
Stand and Deliver (Whole Body) *109*
My Work Here is Done (Whole Body) *111*
Say a Little Prayer (Wrists, Forearms) *113*
Jump To It! (Whole Body) *115*
Dinner Party Diagnosis (General) *117*
Chew On It (Jaw) *119*
Pause for Thought and Boost the Brain (Relaxation, Mobility) *121*
A Note on Stretching (Whole Body) *123*
Add Your Own Exercises *125*
Acknowledgements *129*
About Trish Formby *131*

Foreword

I have been a physio for over thirty years and in this little book I highlight the common issues that have come up repeatedly and I offer simple no-nonsense suggestions to address them.

This is not a heavy book of daunting challenges. The idea is to make staying fit – or tackling a specific issue - easy and fun, without having to leave the home, or break off from your daily schedule and take big chunks out of your day.

Body Fix, Body Fit is a collection of tried-and-tested, evidence-based exercises and approaches that have proved extremely beneficial for many people over many years. I have tried to simplify and describe them to make them quick and straightforward to carry out and to work into a busy daily routine. Follow the ones suitable for you, and the rewards will be sure to follow. Follow them all over a period of time and your body will thank you in the long run.

Leave *Body Fix, Body Fit* lying around to pick up and dip into a few times a day and try the exercise or idea on the page in front of you. Try to stretch yourself – in every sense – and don't just try the ones you recognise or feel most comfortable with! You will feel good in yourself, as well as in your body, for the tiny bit of effort and discipline, and for the pleasing rhythm it will bring to your daily routine. Trust me, I'm a physio!

Trish Formby

"Life isn't a race – you don't want to be the first to finish!"
Trish Formby

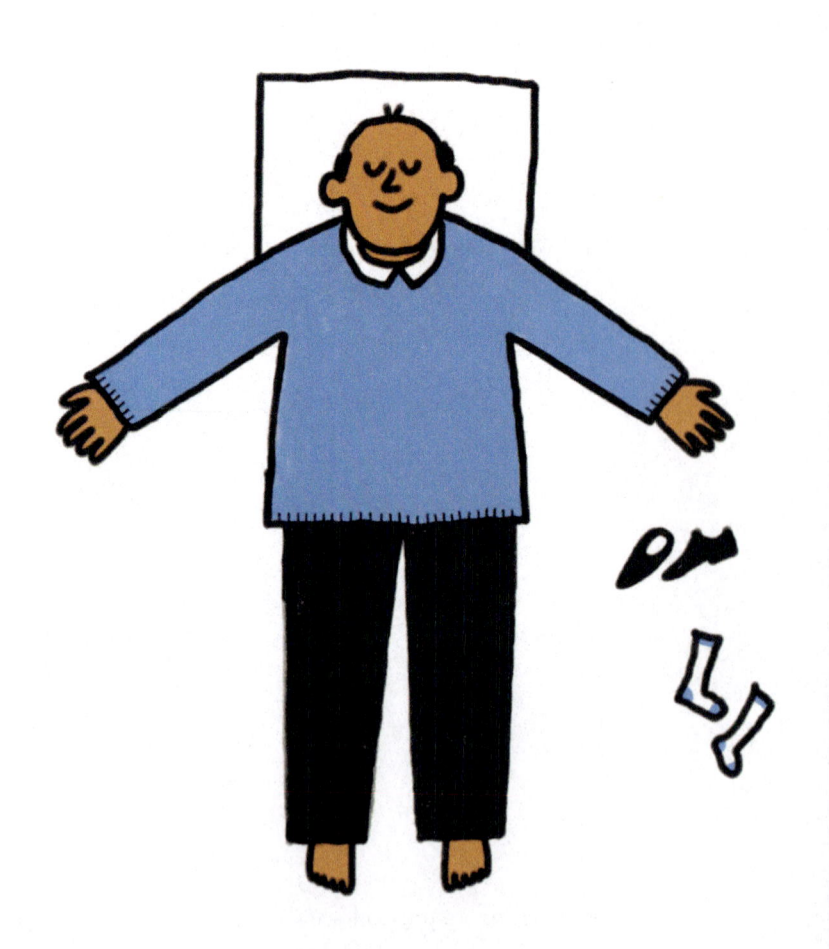

Hit the Reset Button (Relaxation)

Sometimes we need to slow down, pause our busy lives for a moment and hit the reset button. How often do you completely relax during the day? This is a great little exercise for releasing tension.

Lie on your back with your knees bent or straight, whatever feels comfortable. If you can't lie down, sit with your back supported and relax your shoulders. Breathe in through your nose and hold for a few seconds, then exhale slowly letting your diaphragm do the work.

Now try tensing and releasing parts of your body, making sure you completely relax between each contraction. Work through your body from your feet, thighs, bottom, tummy, arms, hands and shoulders until you get to your head. Then open your mouth wide, relax, scrunch your eyes, relax, raise your eyebrow, relax. Now completely relax for a few minutes – are you getting the 'relax' message?! – and enjoy the feeling of the tension leaving your body before getting back to your day.

> Prolonged tension in muscles can be really painful! When our muscles are tensed for long periods the blood vessels get squeezed and the pain receptors become sensitised, which means they fire off pain messages to the brain. Our muscles are hungry for oxygen and this tension prevents them from getting the energy they need and from dumping the waste product.

2 Trish Formby

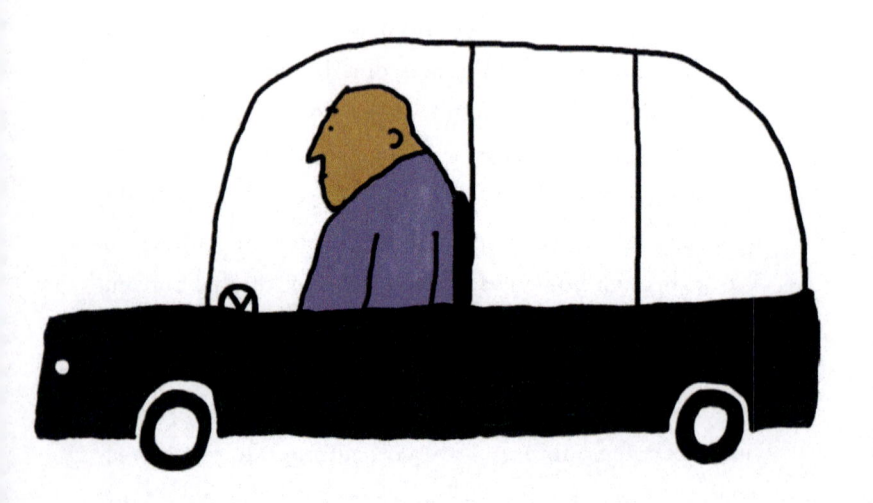

Hit the Floor (Pelvis, Core)

We all have a pelvic floor, the network of sling-like muscles and ligaments that support the organs in your pelvis and contribute to its stability. These are the muscles that control your bladder and bowels. Any dysfunction down there can lead to frequent trips to the loo – and to pain. The good news is you can do your pelvic floor exercises anywhere! They will make a difference.

To contract your pelvic floor, start by relaxing. This is important. Then squeeze your front and back passages together as if stopping yourself from peeing or breaking wind. Try not to squeeze your bottom or inner thigh. Hold that contraction – not that breath (!) – for two seconds and then relax. Repeat 5 to 10 times. Once you have mastered short contractions, try slightly longer ones and work up to 10-second holds.

Try doing your pelvic floor exercises when you are behind the wheel and stopped at traffic lights. If the person in the car next to you has a look of deep concentration and their eyebrows are going up and down, they are probably doing their pelvic floor exercises too!

Caution: don't do your pelvic floor contractions on the loo. This is exactly the time you want your pelvic floor to relax so you can do your business!

4   Trish Formby

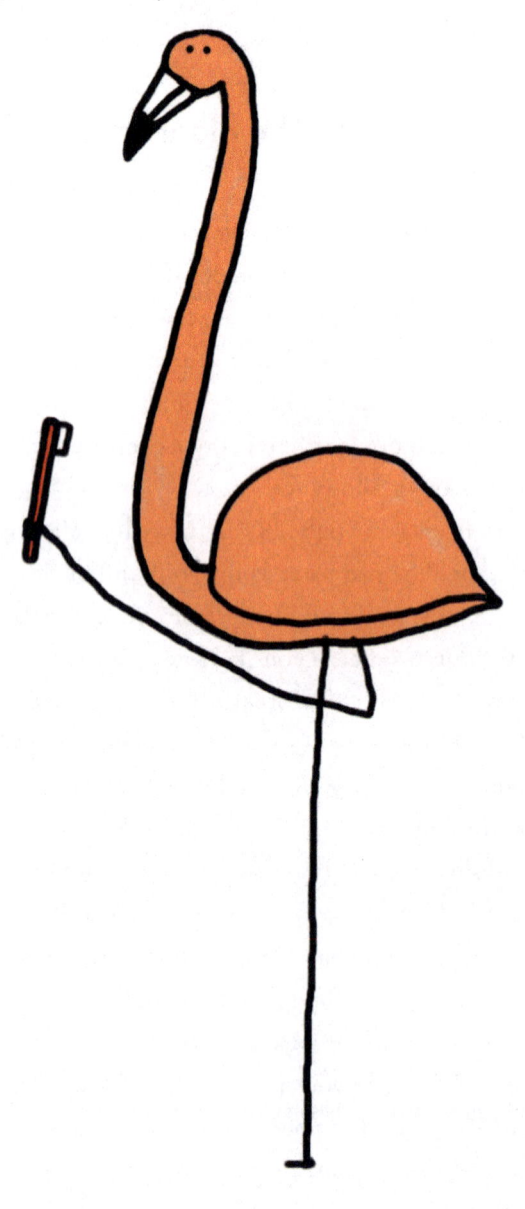

A Leg To Stand On (Balance)

Balance is a skill that often gets worse as we age. The good news is you can improve this crucial function with practice. Balance is achieved through vision, the inner ear and lots of tiny receptors in your muscles and your joints. There can be many reasons for losing balance, but you can improve it by practising little and often.

If your balance is fairly poor, start by standing with your feet apart and transferring your weight from side to side. Slowly lift off one foot at a time and hold. If you are struggling, hold on to something sturdy or put your hands against a wall or surface and gradually reduce the pressure until you can do it without holding. This may take a couple of weeks or so, a few minutes each day, but stick with it. You'll get there.

As you get better, try balancing on one leg for longer. Standing on one leg whilst doing something else, like cleaning your teeth, is a great way to work on your balance. Make sure you try it on both sides. Once you can stand on one leg for a minute or so, make it harder by closing your eyes or increasing the time. Try throwing a ball at a wall or with a friend to make it more challenging (see Child's play).

> Did you know that falls in older people are the cause of around 75,000 hip fractures every year in the UK! These are often caused by a loss of balance. After the age of 65 at least 30 per cent of people fall at least once a year.

6   Trish Formby

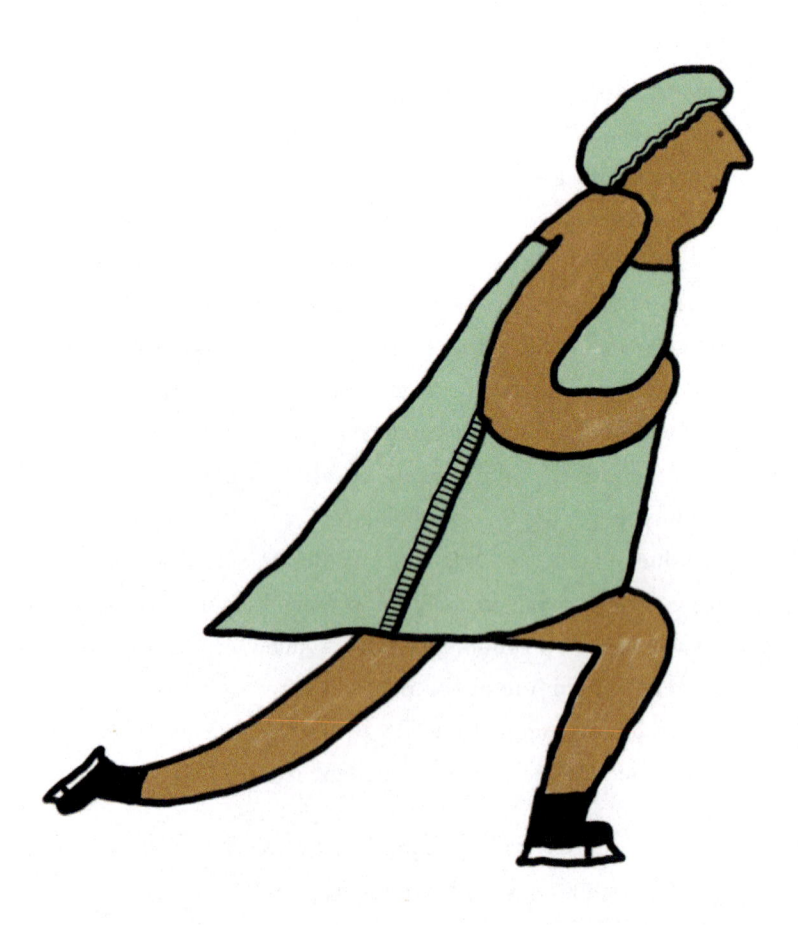

Skating on Thin Ice (Glutes)

The 'Gluteals' are a very important muscle group for pelvic stability and generating force which, in turn, is very important for all sorts of reasons, not least your balance and posture. There are many layers of gluteal muscles but the ones on the outside of the hip are particularly important! Try this simple skating-style exercise to wake them up.

After a shower, place both feet pointing forward on your bathmat, just slightly wider than your shoulder. Bend your knees so you are in a squat position with kneecaps over middle toes. Slide one foot toward the other and away again, then repeat with the other foot until you are skating side to side on the spot. Try doing this for a minute or so and if you fancy working a bit harder try dropping further into the squat.

It is highly unlikely you will ever have to pull on a sequined leotard and perform a Twisting Overhead Lift or Camel Spin, but your body will be grateful for the greater stability and strength.

> There are three large gluteal muscles that all sound like Roman Emperors: gluteus maximus, gluteus minimus and gluteus medius. Beneath these, there are six smaller muscles which control hip lateral rotation and stability of the hip joint.

Trish Formby

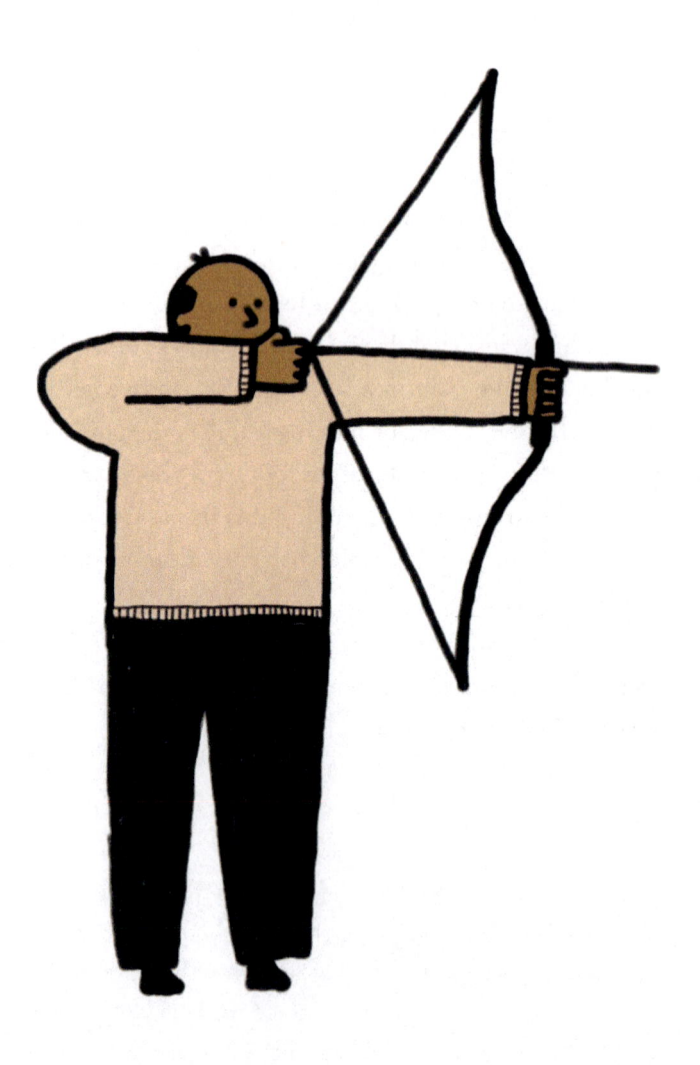

Bow & Arrow (Upper Back)

Rotation of the spine is a really important movement that we use every day. We use it walking, running and in many sports where we are transferring power from our hips and pelvis to our extremities. Any reduction in rotation of the trunk can create more stress in other areas when our body tries to compensate.

Add in some arm movement, and we have not only mobilised the spine but also the shoulders. There are many ways of doing this, the easiest one being the simple act of swinging our arms a little further whilst walking.

Here's a good one when taking a break from the desk and the computer. Start with pointing your arms straight out in front of you, palms together. Slide one hand across the other, down the arm and extend it behind you, leading with the elbow until you look like you are drawing back the arrow of your bow. Keep your eyes focused on the target. Think Sheriff of Nottingham!

If you have long stretchy bands loop them around something sturdy and do the same exercise with a bit of resistance.

> Did you know? They could tell which skeletons were the remains of the bowmen on the wreck of the Mary Rose, Henry VIII's huge warship, from the nobbly bits on the bones of their bowstring arm because they were so much more developed than those on the other crewmen. Given the bows were over six feet long and demanded great strength, that's not surprising!

Trish Formby

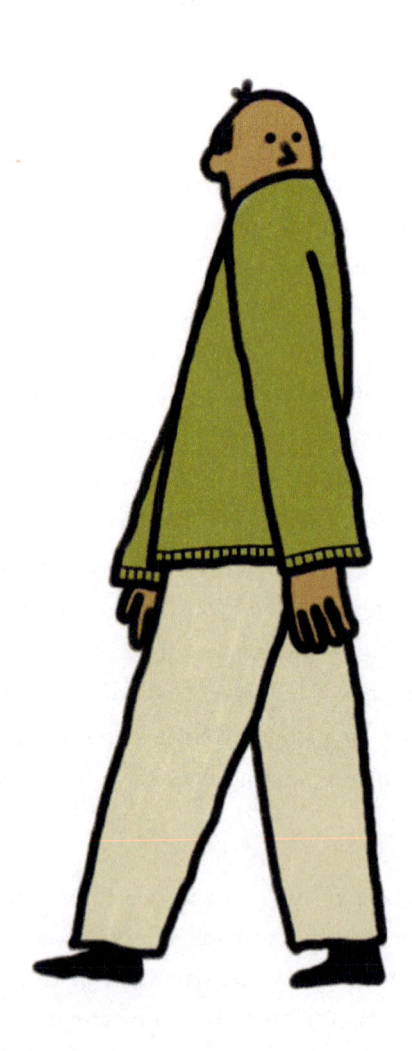

Backtrack (Legs, Brain!)

Walking backwards uses a different muscle action from walking forward and this has been shown to strengthen the ankles and give help to people with arthritis of the knees. Free added bonus: The action also stimulates the brain because it is not familiar with this unusual pattern of movement. Just be careful you are nowhere near a cliff or a swimming pool!

If you have the space, try walking backwards around the dining room table in a clockwise direction and then switch to anticlockwise. As you get better, you can speed up a little and change direction more frequently.

Otherwise, walk backwards in a straight line and then walk forward. Change the speed of these shuttles so you mix up the number of steps, forward and backwards. Go faster as you improve. Try to keep going for a few minutes each session. If you are lucky enough to live near a beach, try walking backwards on the sand. Ignore the strange looks!

Trish Formby

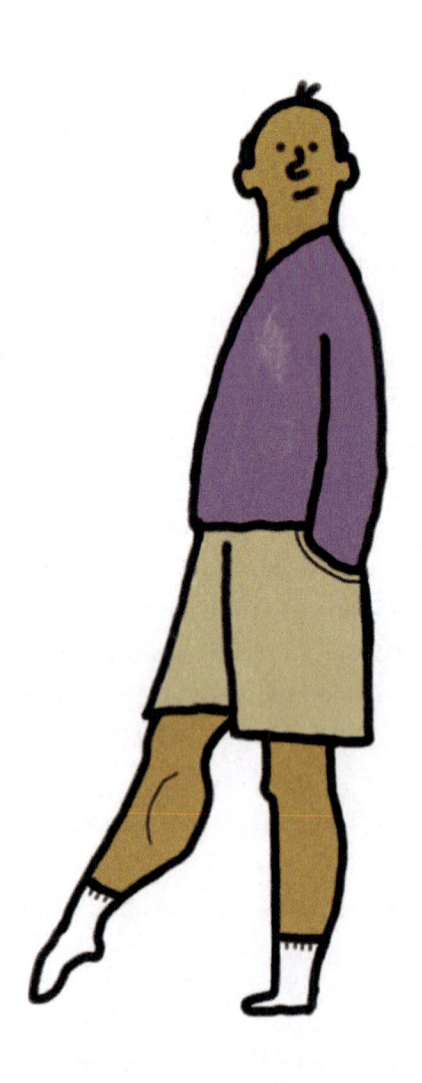

All Rise (Calves)

Your calves are the power muscles that assist push-off during walking, running, jumping and hopping. They also provide stability at the ankle and knee joints. It's a really important muscle group and one that often gets overlooked.

Every time you go upstairs or steps, try doing five to ten calf raises. Start on the lowest step with your heels hanging over the back and hold on lightly to the banister. Rise onto your toes as high as you can go then lower the back of the foot until your heels are below the level of the step. Repeat ten times slowly on both legs.

Once you can do ten repetitions comfortably, try doing it on one leg and keep increasing the number as far as you can. You can vary it on the stairs by choosing a different step every time or try rising onto your toes every step as you climb.

It all depends on your age, but you should be able to do 20 to 30 repetitions of a calf raise on each leg up to your late 60s, and 10 to 20 reps after the age of 70.

Achilles tendinopathy is the condition of weakened and degenerate collagen reacting to overload. This may be the result of taking up a new sport, increasing jogging or running mileage too quickly or suddenly introducing hill climbs into your runs. In these instances your body may not have had time to adapt to the new stresses. Many people try to 'stretch out the pain' but it is best treated with this progressive regime of calf raises as they will stimulate collagen production.

14 Trish Formby

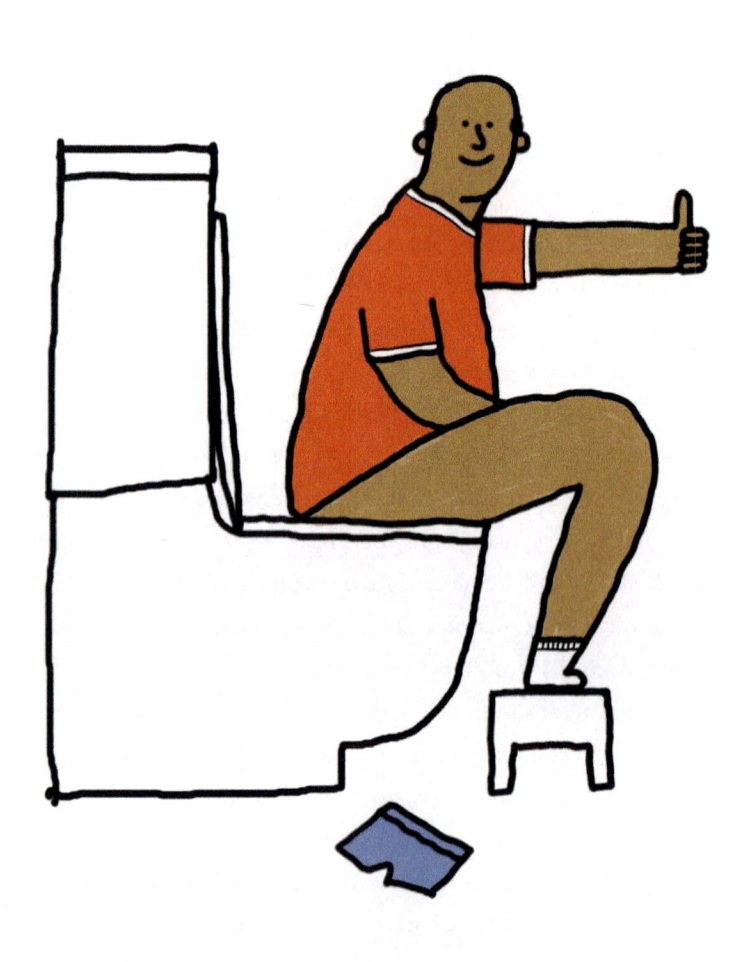

Super Pooper Trooper (Bowels)

Did you know that if you put a small step under your feet whilst you sit on the toilet it will help you poop? Doing this allows gravity to work its magic by placing your pelvis in the correct position so that the colon is straightened, and your line of fire is better! It is similar to the squatting position but with less effort on the legs.

Place a small stool under your feet so your knees are slightly higher than your hip and your feet are flat, then lean slightly forward. You should not force your bowel movement or strain but if you are having difficulty in this area, make sure you are drinking enough water, taking some fibre in your diet and getting some exercise.

Most women have a slightly longer colon than men. This means it takes a little longer for food to pass through their digestive tract and can make them more prone to bloating, so plenty of fibre is even more important!!

16   Trish Formby

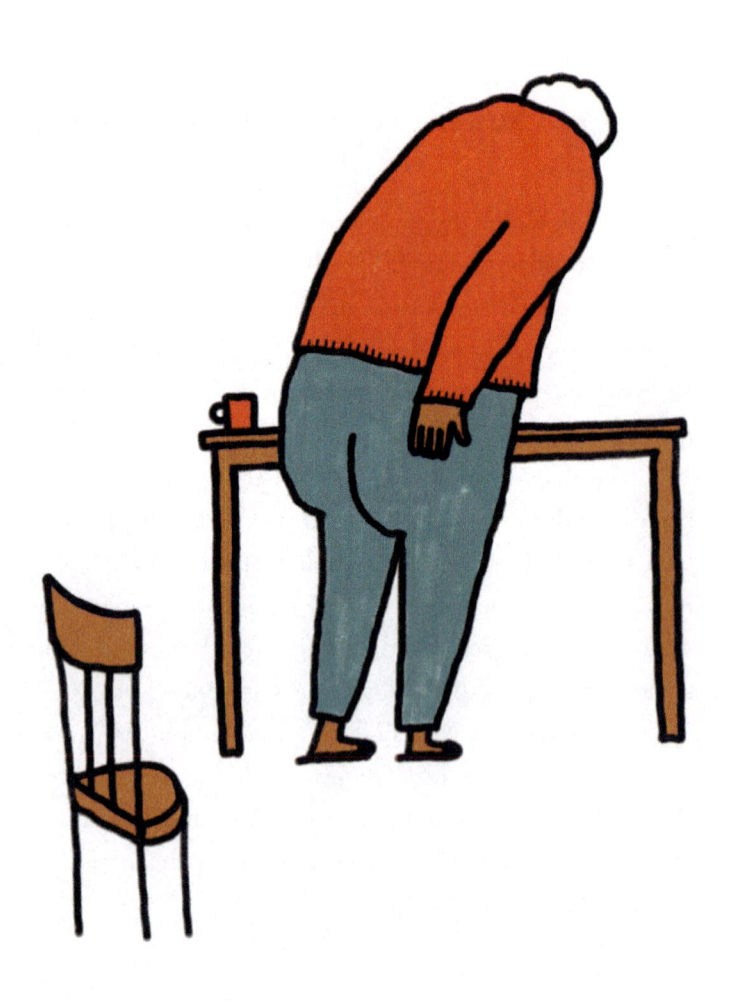

Get off Your Butt! (Glutes)

The gluteus maximus muscles (your buttocks) are the largest and strongest in your body and they see a lot of action. We use them all the time, most often during push-off to extend our hips while walking and running. Scientists say that the reason we can walk so well on two legs is most likely a result of our large butts. The problem is that instead of running across the plains of Africa as our ancestors might have, we spend most of our time sitting on it! The modern human therefore needs to give their butt special attention.

A quick way of firing up your gluteus maximus is to stand a couple of feet facing away from a wall. Bend one knee to ninety degrees and place your foot on the wall behind you. Now really squeeze your butt and push yourself away from the wall. Keep squeezing for 30 seconds. Now repeat on the other leg.

If you want a tougher challenge, try bending and straightening the supporting leg like a single-leg squat or try rising onto your toes. Make sure you keep your kneecap over your middle toe if you go into a bend.

18   Trish Formby

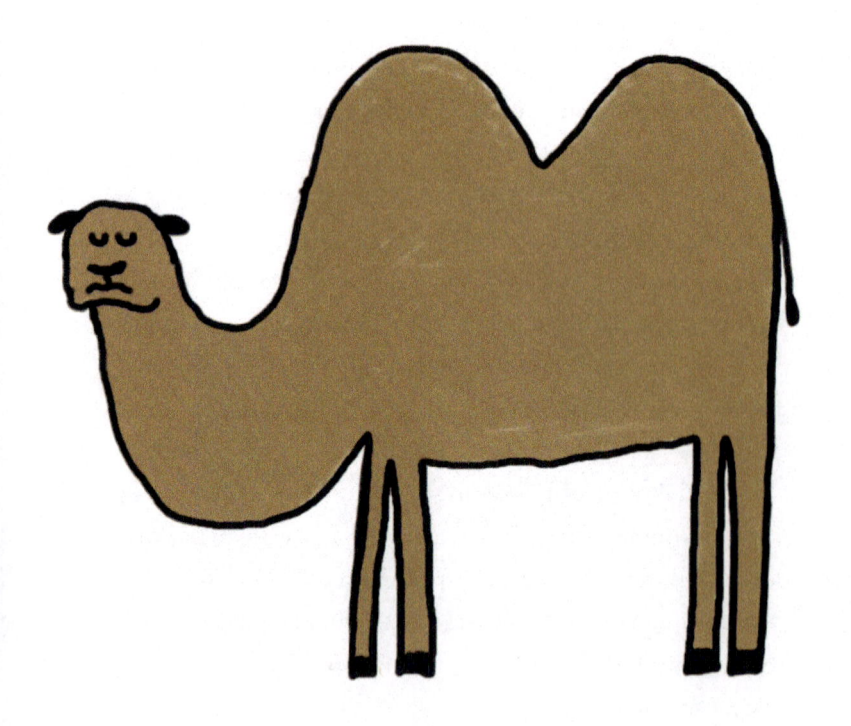

Don't get the Hump (Upper Back)

The very upper part of our back, just below the neck, can become very stiff and cause all sorts of problems. This has become more of an issue in recent times, the result of our heads craning forward over computers or smartphones. These positions cause increased tension in the muscles spanning your neck and shoulders and in turn, the joints at the top of the back can stiffen or even seize up.

Try mobilising this area by stretching over a bolster (a log-shaped pillow, foam roller or rolled towel), an inflatable exercise ball or even over the armrest of a sofa. If you look around, you can find lots of features around the house that will work. Position yourself so that whatever you are stretching over is between your shoulder blades.

Support your head by clasping your hands behind your neck and bringing your chin ever so slightly to your chest, then stretch backwards using your bolster as a fulcrum. Keep your head supported so that the movement is in your upper back not your neck – then breathe out a happy sigh. Follow up with **Bow and Arrow** and you're set for another bout at your desk or a game of tennis

20 Trish Formby

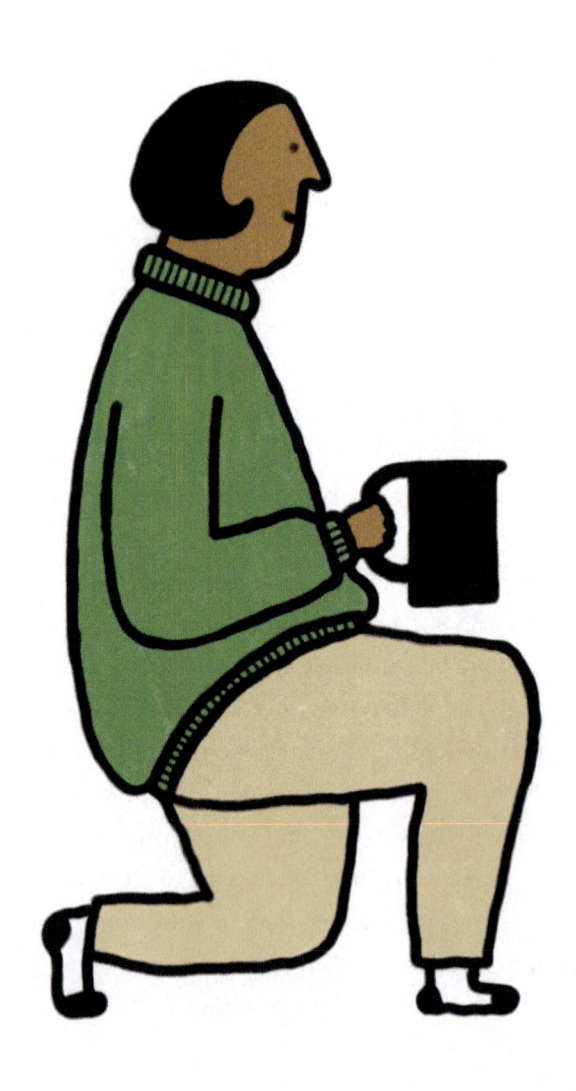

Ministry of Funny Walks (Lower Body, Core)

Maybe don't give it the full Monty Python but, like backwards walking, varying your walk forces you to use different muscles and different brain patterns as well as strengthening and mobilising different parts of the body. When we walk, we use a little trunk rotation and arm swing but, unless you're a tip-toeing house burglar, we don't go through massive ranges of motion in the lower part of our body.

Try walking on your toes or walking on your heels when you go to make a cup of tea – or, if you're feeling skittish, you could try the famous Groucho Marx walk. For those too young to remember the comedian, this is walking with your knees really bent and as low to the ground as you can.

Another good one is to start with the feet wide apart and drop down into a squat. Now walk sideways like a crab always leading with the same leg. Don't forget to lead with the other leg on the way back.

Or, try a Cossack Dance where you lunge forward in the squat position with the arms crossed at shoulder height. As you lunge forward onto the right leg, twist your body to the right, then repeat with a left lunge and so on. Keep moving forward (or sideways)– you'll get to the kettle eventually and enjoy your tea all the more!

Trish Formby

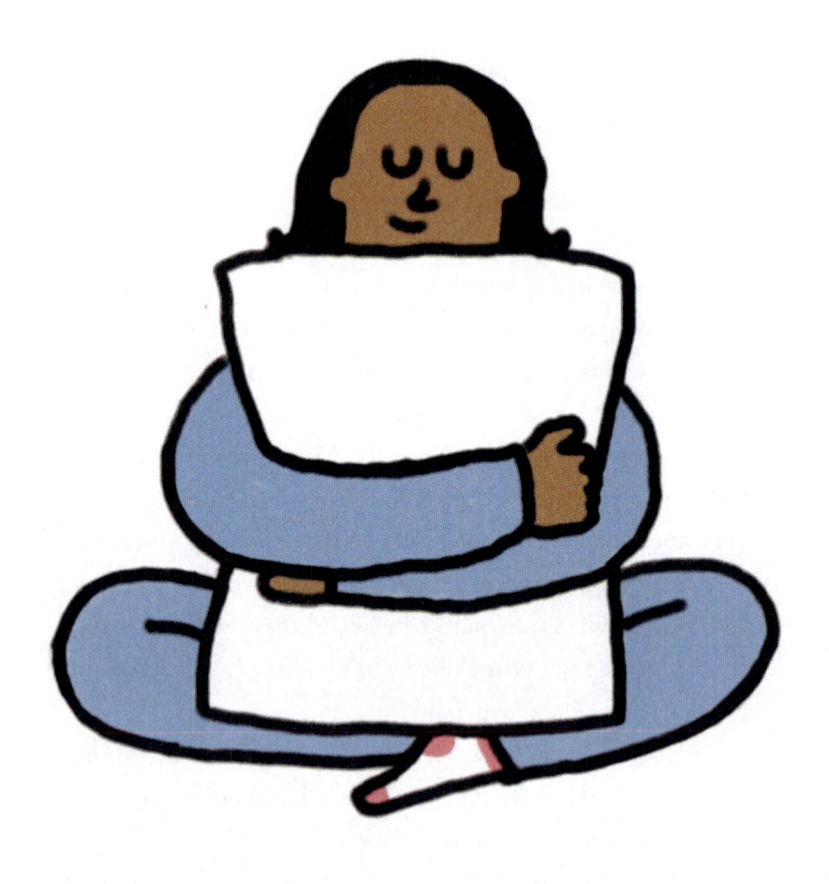

Pillow Talk (Sleep Comfort)

It can be difficult to find a pillow suitable for the way we sleep. There are so many different types of filling that it is almost impossible to know what is right for you until you have slept on it. However, there are some general rules of thumb that you can follow.

If you are someone who sleeps on your back, then you want a pillow that keeps your head and neck pretty much in line with your spine. Some people need a little more support under the curve of the neck so having a feather pillow that you can plump up in this area can help, or a firmer pillow with an inbuilt ridge.

If you sleep on your side, you might need a slightly plumper pillow or even two pillows to allow for the width of your shoulders. Be careful you don't go too high. You still want to keep your neck in line with your body and again, you might want extra support in the neck area.

If you suffer from back pain, try placing a pillow between your knees when lying on your side. This will keep your pelvis square. If you suffer from shoulder pain, you might want to cuddle a pillow in front of you.

Sleeping on your tummy is not the best position, although many people do. If you suffer from neck pain, it's probably best not to. Try instead to sleep with a pillow in front of you so you quarter-turn toward your tummy and gradually train yourself out of it.

24 Trish Formby

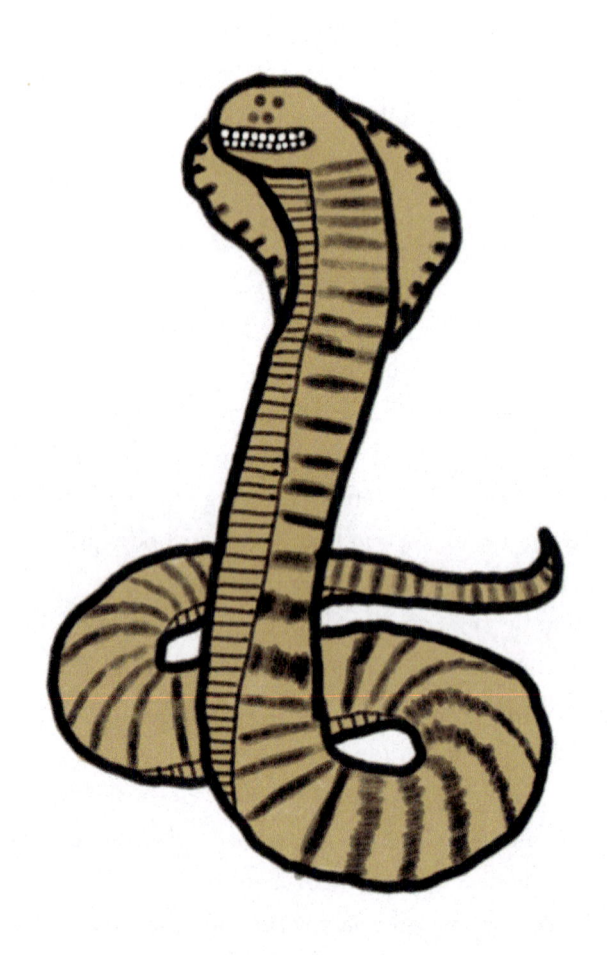

Rear like a Cobra (Back Extension)

If you have been sitting all day or doing a lot of chores that require you to bend forward, you might want to reverse the position from time to time. The 'cobra' is just such a movement, named after the deadly darting snake, that rears up when threatened.

If you can, lie on the floor on your tummy. Place your hands flat on the floor to the side of your head level with your ears. Now push onto your hands keeping your back nice and relaxed. Make sure you keep your hips on the floor and push up to where it feels comfortable. Lower yourself down and then raise again. If it feels comfortable you can push up a little higher each time. Repeat 5 times.

> Snakes have between 300 and 400 vertebrae and they have a pair of ribs attached to each one. Compare that to our paltry 33 vertebrae (including 9 fused bones in the sacrum and coccyx) and 12 pairs of ribs. Apparently, snakes can have back pain too so spare a thought.... unless it's rearing up at you!

26   Trish Formby

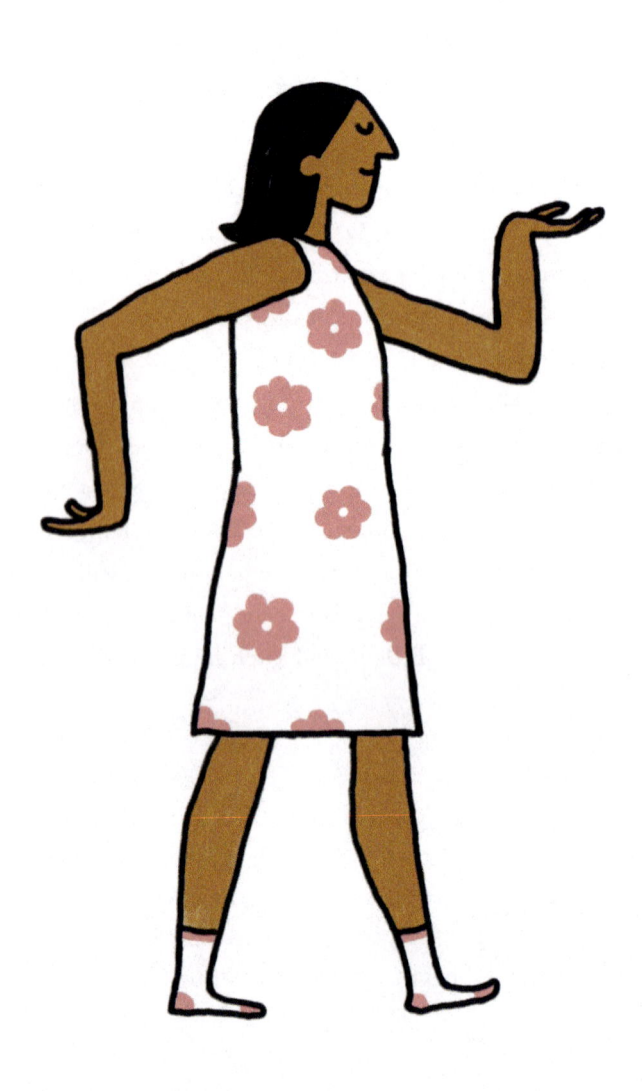

Walk like an Egyptian (Shoulders)

Does this really need an explanation? The iconic image of an Egyptian with one arm bent at ninety degrees and the palm up to the ceiling and the other bent downward at ninety degrees and the palm still up to the ceiling is well known. There's even a song about it! You've probably done it on the dancefloor after a few too many.

This routine will mobilise your shoulders. Stand with your feet slightly apart or even with your back supported against a wall. Take your arms out to the side to shoulder height with your palms facing forward and bend your elbows to ninety degrees, keeping your shoulders wide. Now rotate one arm downwards toward the horizontal whilst keeping the other arm up and then reverse. Do not force the movement or try to go beyond a comfortable position. If you find it difficult to hold your arm up then try resting your elbow on a surface and do one arm at a time. You can add in light weights 1-2kg so long as you can control the movement and you have no pain.

> Egyptians didn't actually walk like this – who would have thought? Our ancient ancestors from the Nile Delta are depicted like this because artists drew in two dimensions only, representing each part of the body in its most recognisable form.

Trish Formby

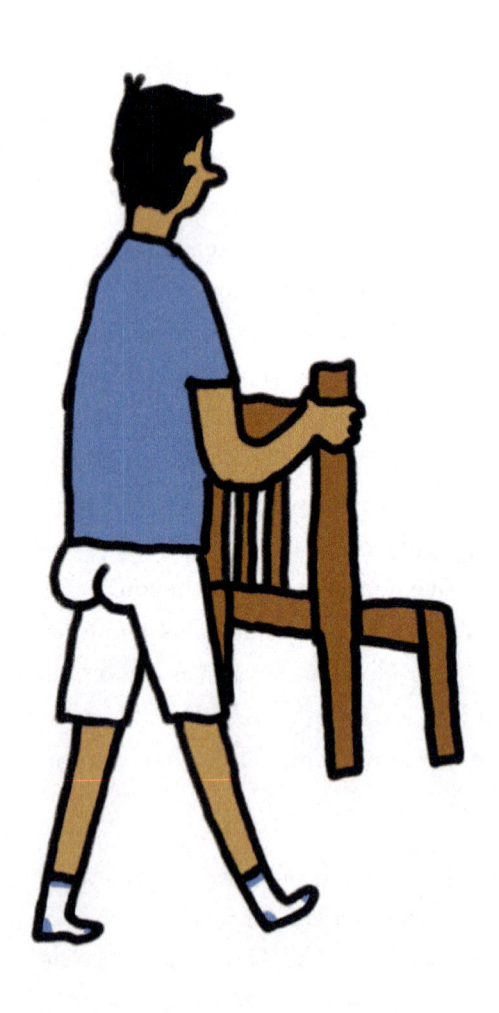

Bridge the Gap (Thighs, Bums and Tums)

'Bridging' is a fantastic exercise for achieving a pert behind and it also works your thighs, bottom and tummy so it's great for pelvic stability too.

Lie on your back and bend your knees to ninety degrees with your feet flat on the floor. Lift your bottom off the floor, hold for a couple of seconds and then lower down. Repeat ten times.

There are many variations that you can try with this exercise. For a change, try placing your feet on a wall so that your hips and knees are both bent to ninety degrees and your feet are shoulder-width apart. Lift your bottom from that position and hold or repeat ten times. Give an extra squeeze of your butt when you get to the top.

Or you can put your feet on a chair and lift your bottom. This will engage the hamstrings at the back of the thigh a bit more.

Trish Formby

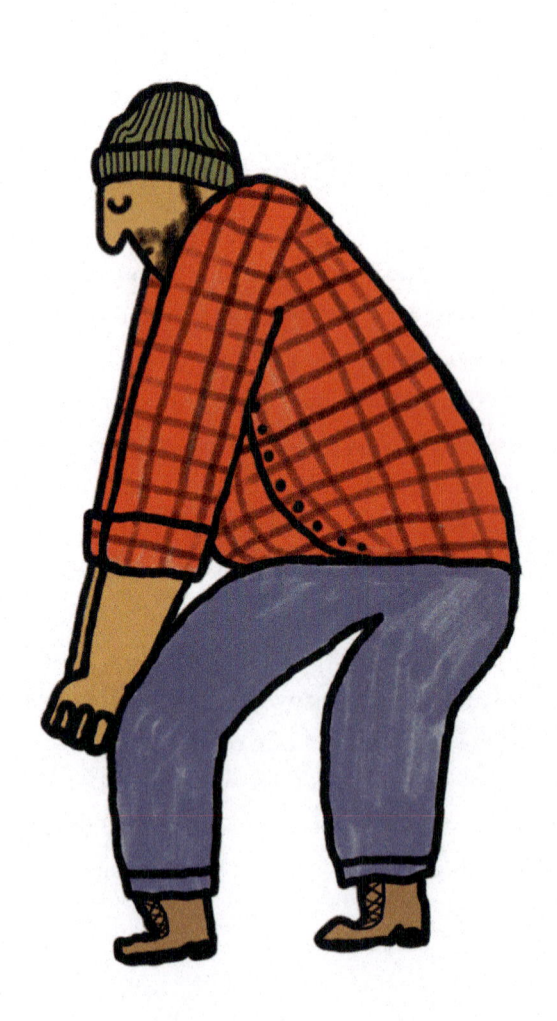

Wood Chop (Whole Body, Functional)

This is a brilliant exercise that combines the stability of the pelvis and lower limbs with mobility of the trunk and upper limb. It's the strategy that we use to generate and conserve energy when playing sports. It uses the concept of conservation of momentum where the larger stronger segments generate a rotational force which is then transferred smoothly through the kinetic chain out to our extremities to generate speed for things like hitting a ball or throwing an object.

Start with your feet slightly wider than your hips. Clasp your hands in front of you. Now squat down and take your hands to your right knee. As you straighten up rotate to your left and extend your arms, hands still clasped, upwards and over your left shoulder. Then return back to the right knee. Repeat 10 times and then do the other side. To progress this exercise, you can do this holding a light weight with both hands or a weighted ball. Keep the movement smooth.

> Did you know studies have shown that just over 50% of the power in a professionals tennis serve is generated by the trunk and the legs and the rest is a combination of shoulder, elbow and wrist.

Trish Formby

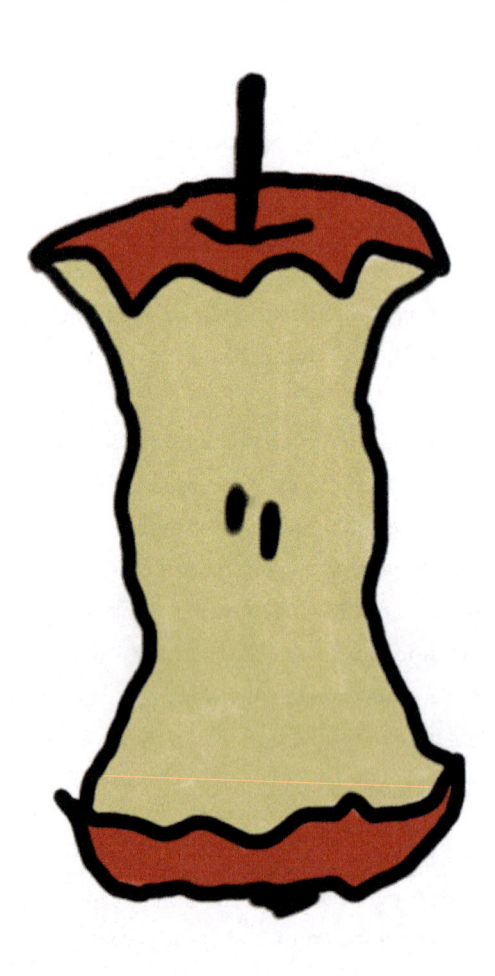

Core Blimey (Core)

People talk about the 'core' all the time without really ever explaining what it is or how it works. We usually refer to the core as being the muscles around our pelvis and spine but actually, all of our joints have their own version of a core.

Quite simply, we have two systems of muscles in our body, described as our local and global systems.

The muscles of the local system are close to the joints and, in the case of the spine, span just a few segments. These muscles help to control movement and make small adjustments to support our joints and make sure they run smoothly.

The global system is a second network of muscles that tend to be further away from the joint axis, often longer, or spanning more than one segment. These muscles are the ones that create movement at a joint or even two or three joints.

So, there we have it. The 'core' muscles, or local system, control movement and the global system creates movement. They work in synergy and the most important thing is that they are balanced … but you could write a whole book about that. Please don't make me do that.

34 Trish Formby

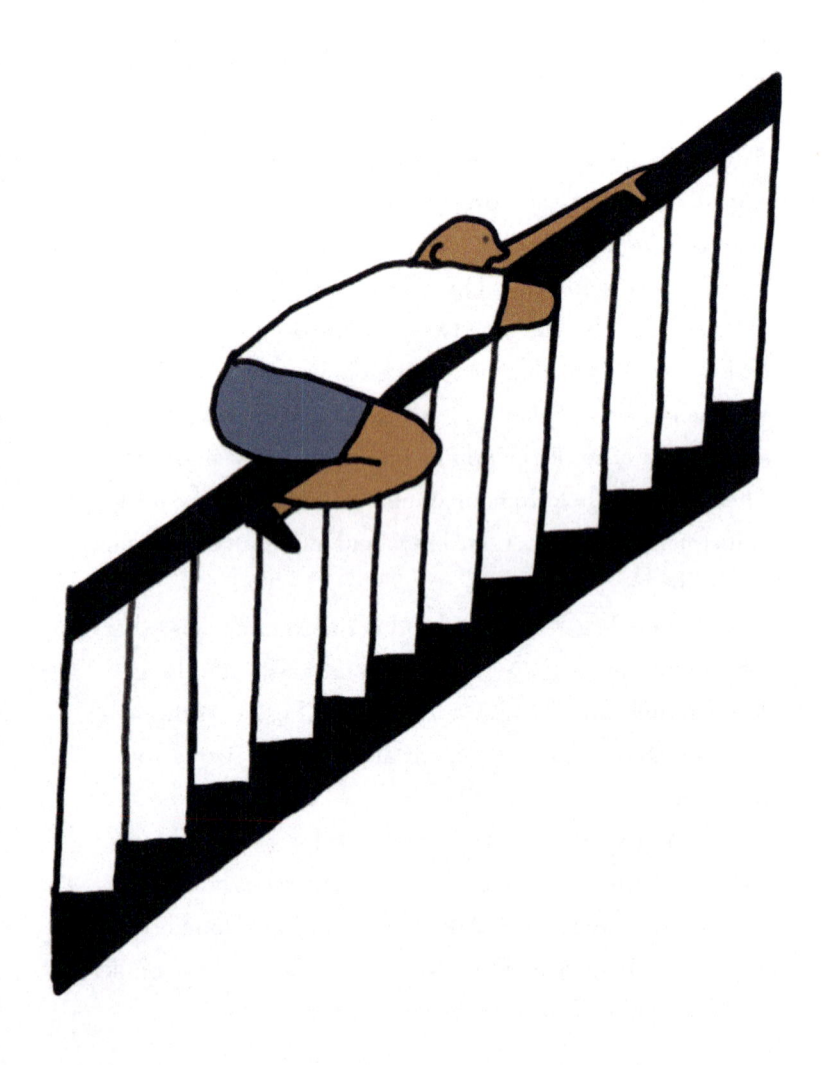

Don't Wait for an Emergency to Take the Stairs (Whole Body)

I hate lifts because I get claustrophobic in small spaces but that's not the only reason I take the stairs. Taking the stairs has so many health benefits that I must list them.

- When you climb stairs, you are taking 3 to 4 times your body weight, so it is a great way of strengthening the quads and gluteals
- Stair-climbing uses 8 to 11 kcal per minute
- Stair-climbing is essentially a resistance exercise, so it is great for helping with bone density
- Climbing two flights of stairs per day can contribute to losing 2.7kg of weight per year
- Using the stairs will enhance your circulation and your lung capacity and it has been shown to lower cholesterol when done regularly

So, next time you see that little sign pointing to the stairs, ditch the lift and the escalators and take the more active route whenever you can.

36 Trish Formby

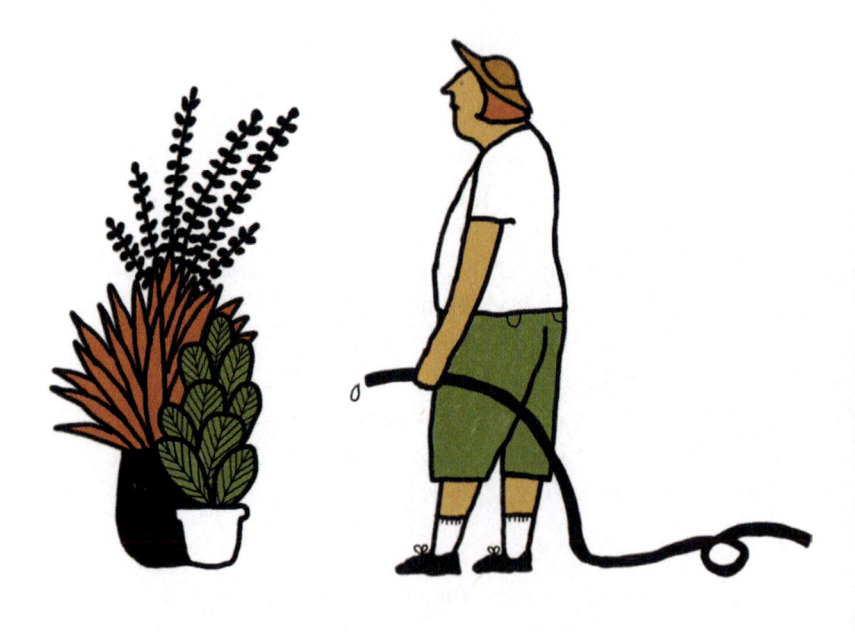

The Gardener's Joy... and Pain (Lower Back, Knees)

Gardening brings great joy to many people, but it can also bring intense or chronic pain. Leaning forward over flowerbeds, bending to pot plants, weeding, working the push mower – that's a lot of repetitive and sustained load on the lower back. Gardeners often feel some back and neck pain, or stiffness after a long day with the secateurs, trowel and watering can. Kneeling for long periods can also cause pain in the front of the knee.

Try mixing up the tasks, take regular breaks from repetitive tasks, and, where possible, stand upright or take one knee to pot plants or weeding. Every now and then, stand up, place your hands on your hips and stretch backwards to reverse the bent-over position. Use a foam cushion to kneel on if you must get down low and – I repeat! – be sure to take regular breaks from all prolonged activities.

Make sure you use a harness if holding a strimmer or hedge trimmer to take the weight. This will distribute the load, and it is also much safer! Do not try to lift anything too heavy for you. Either get help or invest in a small trolley if you need to move heavy objects around the garden.

When you finish, do an exercise or two from this book, then sit back and enjoy the rewards of all your efforts.

38 Trish Formby

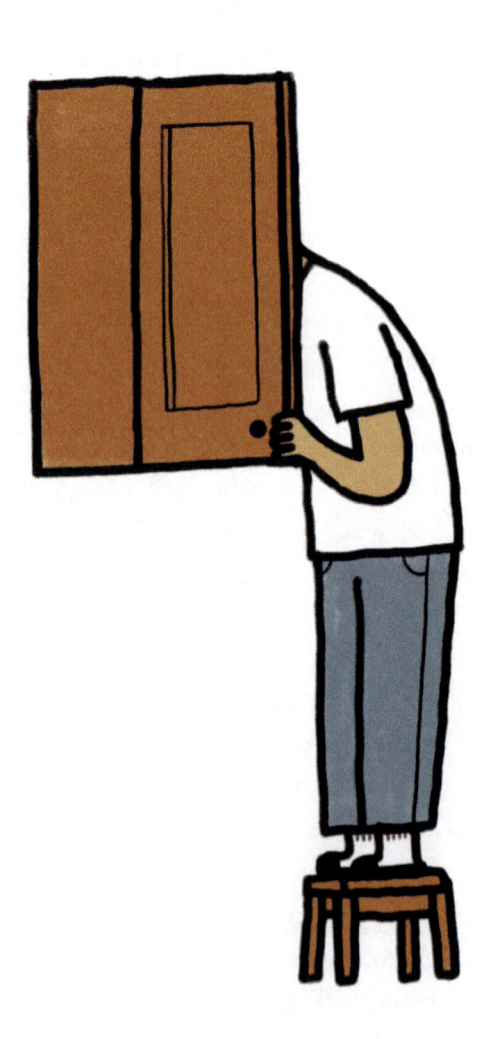

DIY stands for Don't Injure Yourself (Whole Body)

Apart from the obvious injuries like hitting your thumb with a hammer, there are also many varieties of repetitive strain injuries caused by DIY, particularly in the shoulders, elbows and wrists. Painting ceilings and walls … hammering… sanding … lifting …

In fact, tennis and golfer 'elbows' are not always caused by these sports. The problem is often the result of intensive DIY. You might not feel it in the moment, but the pain or aches will come overnight or the next day. If you are carrying out sustained DIY tasks over a few days, you might find that the pain becomes excruciating. Trust me! I've been there and I take strict measures to avoid it.

To reduce the risk of RSI and other injuries, try to get yourself in a good position. Use a sturdy step stool for overhead tasks and a kneeling pad for tasks close to the floor. Try to use your leg muscles when scrubbing or vacuuming to take the strain from your arms. Make sure you take regular breaks and vary the tasks. During breaks try some of the pause exercises in this book. **Pass the Baton and Don't Get the Hump** are good ones for many DIY tasks.

Make sure you give yourself plenty of recovery time too. Often, it's the accumulation of repetitive tasks that causes the problems.

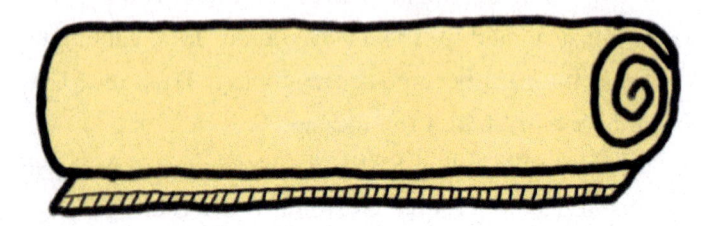

Throw the Towel In
(Back, Neck, Breathing)

Look around the house and you will find many common items that can be used as part of your daily exercise and stretching routines. Towels are particularly versatile, and this is one of my favourites!

Make a small log by folding a hand towel into thirds and rolling it into a cylindrical shape. Then place a pillow on the floor with the rolled towel perpendicular, so it creates a T-shape. Lie on your back with your head on the pillow, the towel running up your spine and your shoulder blades falling on either side.

This a great rest position if you have been sitting or driving and want to stretch out for a few minutes and it is also a good starting position for breathing and neck exercises such as **Take a Breather** or **Hit the Reset Button**.

42   Trish Formby

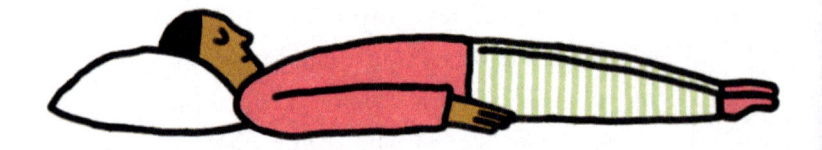

Chin Up, Old Boy (Neck, Shoulders)

Actually, it is more chin down. Often, as we get tired from working in one position and our postural neck muscles become fatigued, we begin to slouch and adopt a 'poked chin'. Over time, this creates strain on the shoulder and neck muscles so it's very important to take regular short breaks.

Lie down on your back with a rolled towel and a pillow as per **Throw The Towel In**. Start by breathing through your nose deep into your lower ribs, whilst keeping your shoulders relaxed. Gently drop your chin downward as if nodding and press lightly into the pillow.

Imagine making your neck longer. Make sure you keep the muscles at the front of your neck relaxed. Feel them – they should be soft. Hold this position for three slow breaths in and out.

After a few repetitions, roll your head to the left and the right, keeping a little pressure through the base of your skull and making sure you keep the chin slightly down whilst lengthening at the back of the neck.

44   Trish Formby

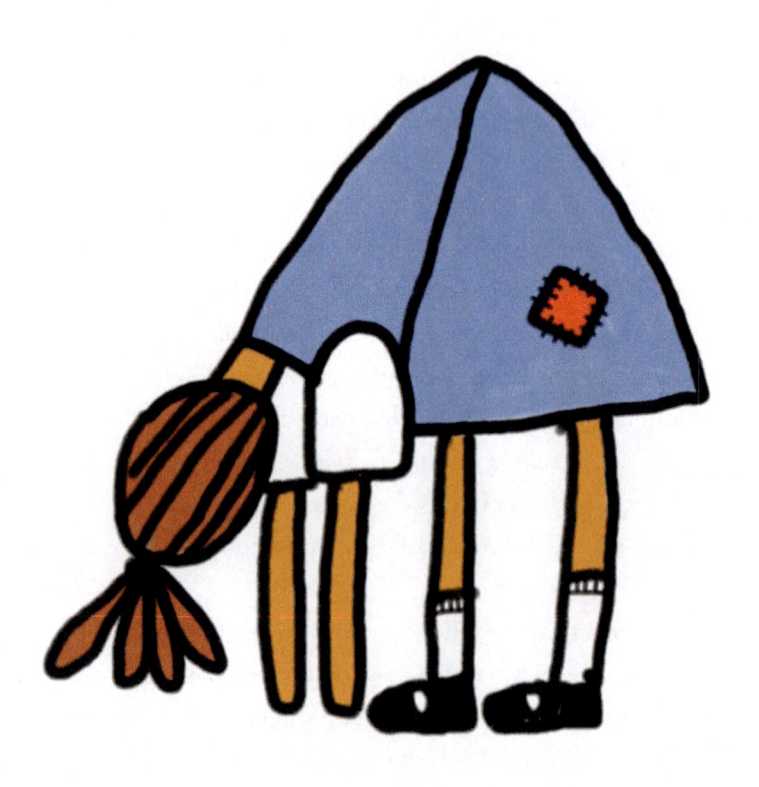

Roll Up! Roll Up! (Back)

Bending forward – or flexion of the spine – is a normal movement but many people are wary of bending because they have been told that it is not good for them. If you stop bending, you will likely become stiff and begin to brace in your lower back. This creates strain on the muscles, alters breathing patterns and can cause abnormal movement patterns.

If you are a little anxious about bending your spine, start by standing with your back against a wall and your feet about two feet away from it and shoulder-width apart. Start by taking a breath in and, as you exhale, begin to roll down, firstly by taking your chin to your chest. Now slide your hands down the front of your thigh, trying to curl your spine until you are hanging like a ragdoll with your knees slightly bent. Only go as far as you feel comfortable.

When you get to the bottom, take another breath in and start to roll your way back up. Imagine you are scooping your belly button toward your spine as you roll up, then return to standing with your back supported by the wall. Repeat 2 or 3 times.

46 Trish Formby

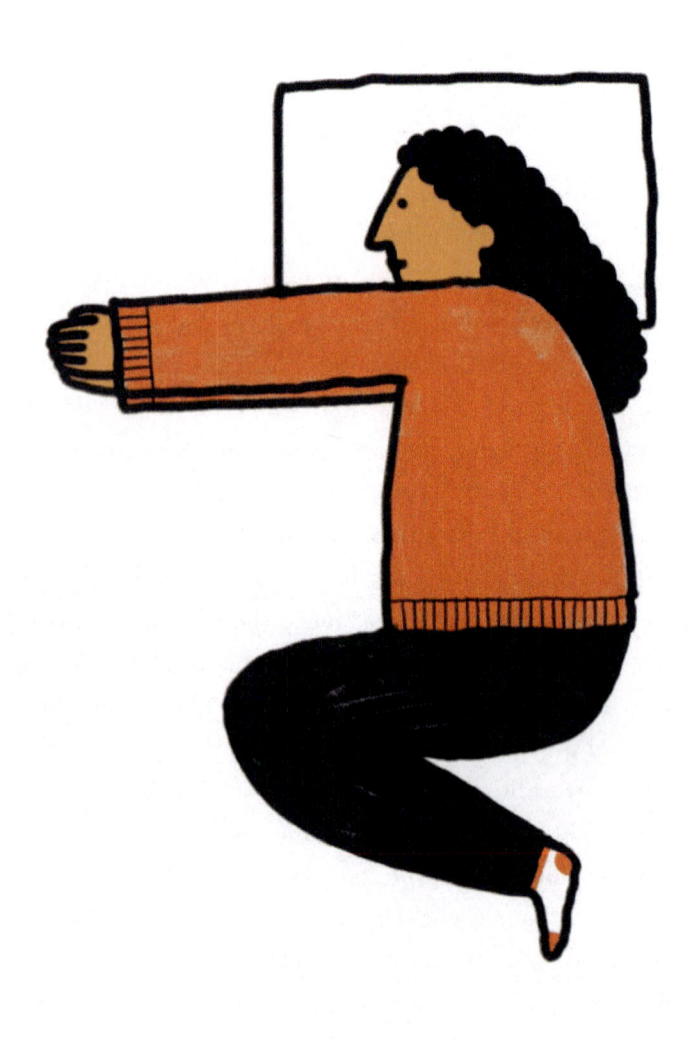

Make That Trunk Call (Back, Arms)

Keeping your upper back mobile is very important. This little gem adds in some arm movement so you get a nice stretch across the front of your shoulder and, because you are lying down it is very relaxing.

Start by lying on your side with a pillow under your head and your knees bent. Place your arms straight out in front with the palms together. Now slide the top palm over the bottom arm and then across your chest, whilst allowing your trunk to roll back and turn your head to follow the arm.

Once you reach the shoulder, begin to extend the arm and stretch it out behind you. Only take the arm as far as you are comfortable, then bring it back to the starting position by reversing all the movements. Repeat a few times and then roll over and do the same on the other side.

When we mobilise in any direction we are also mobilising our nervous system. Nerves need to be able to slide and glide through the body and exercises like this one for the upper limb can be helpful but should not be painful. Our nervous system is one continuous complex system which allows our brain to communicate with the rest of the body. If you were to add up all the nerves in the body, it would be more than 45 miles long!

48 Trish Formby

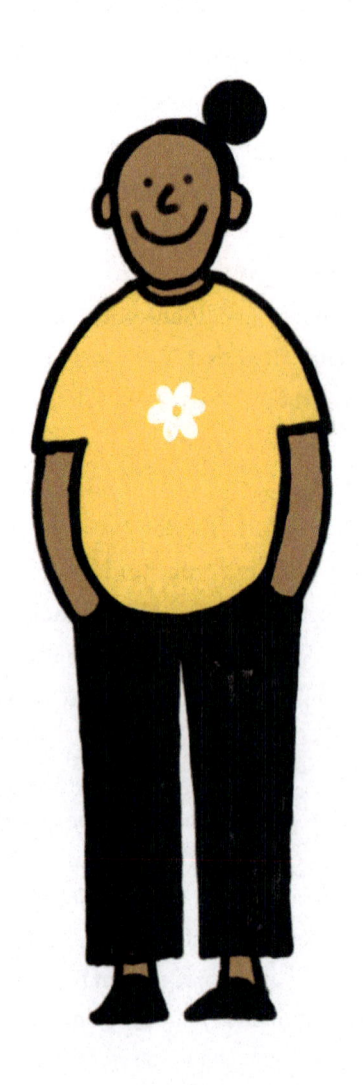

Go on, Give Us a Smile (Happiness!)

No really, just smile! Except maybe if you're at a funeral.

Smiling can boost your mood and the mood of those around you. Smiling has been shown to reduce stress and release happy hormones. Not only that, but people also tend to smile back so you get a double boost to the mood. Buy into a smile, get one free!

Even if you don't feel like it, try smiling right now. You might even find yourself laughing at what you're doing. Who's watching?

It takes more muscles to frown than it does to smile so it's actually less work than being grumpy. Smiling is known to reduce cortisol, the stress hormone, and, smile by smile, it strengthens the immune system. And if that doesn't make you smile…

Trish Formby

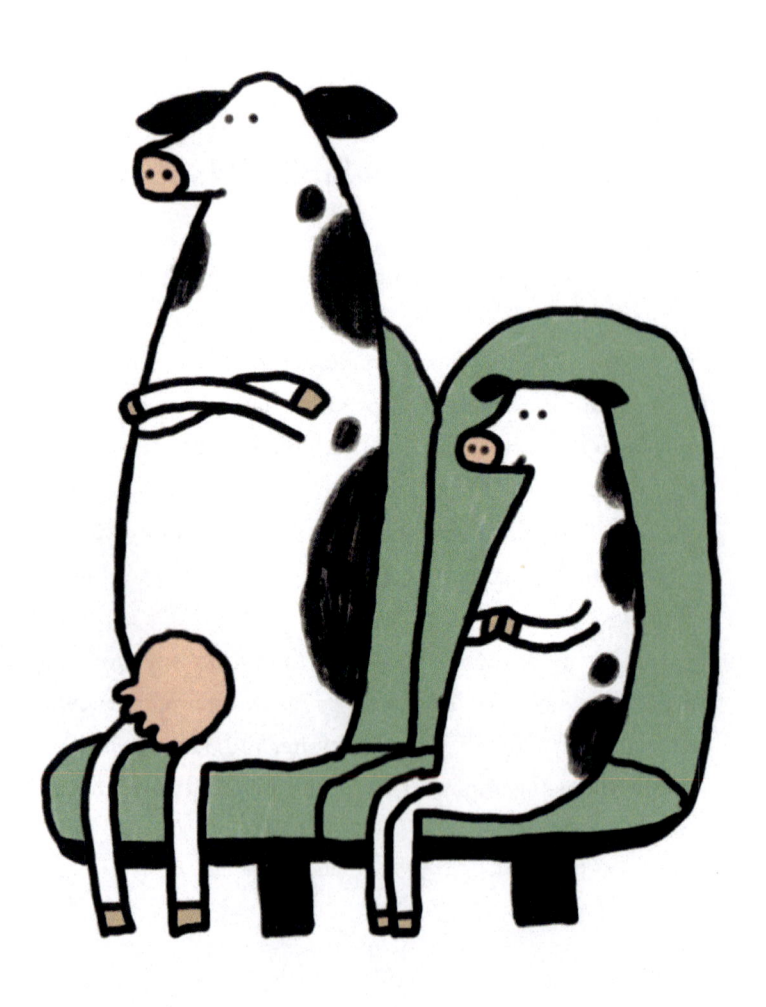

Bent Knee Calf Raise (Calf)

Calf raises with bent knees make the deeper part of the muscle work a bit harder. The 'soleus' is a very important muscle that we use for pushing off and stabilising the ankle. It also plays the crucial role of pumping blood back to the heart against gravity, working to keep our circulation flowing when we are standing or sitting.

Here's a neat little exercise to keep the soleus happy. Stand with your feet slightly apart and lower into a squat position. Now rise onto your toes keeping down low in the squat.

If you are sitting for a long time, say on a flight or a train, you can do this in your seat – and make sure you do plenty of them to keep your circulation going. For a separate little stretch, try keeping your heels down and lifting and splaying your toes.

> Deep vein thrombosis is a dangerous condition where a blood clot forms, most commonly in the calves and thighs, affecting 1-2 per 1,000 people every year. The main causes include post-surgery recovery, immobilisation and obesity. Travelling by car, train or plane for more than 4 hours can double the risk of thrombosis. Do those calf raises to reduce the risk.

52 Trish Formby

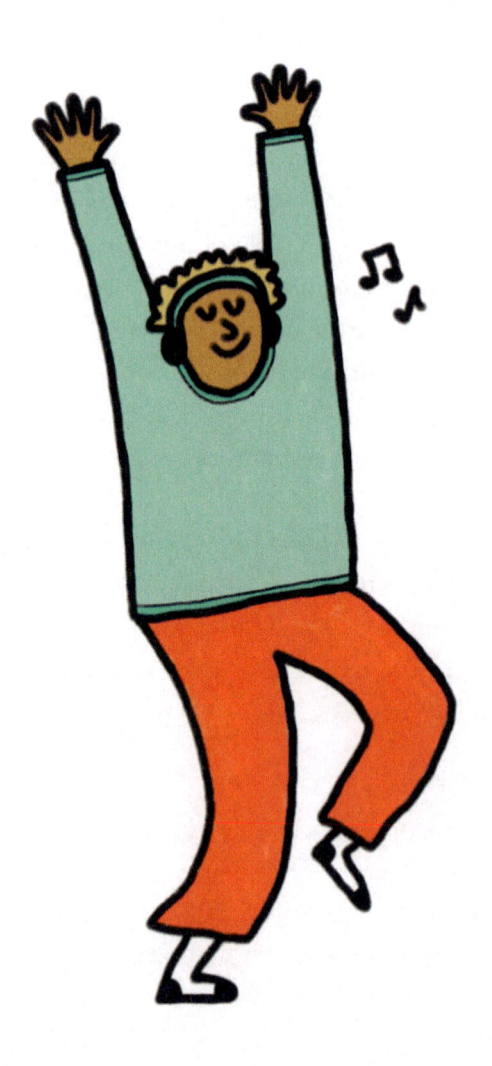

Kitchen Disco (Cardio)

People have been dancing since pre-historic times. Cave drawings in India, the earliest records, show people getting down and grooving ten thousand years ago. Way back in the day, dancing tended to be associated with religious rituals and ceremonies; in modern times it has become more of a pure entertainment, bringing people together to express their culture and celebrate happy events.

Dancing has proven health benefits: improving cardiovascular fitness, increasing flexibility and firing up the happy hormones, boosting your mood as you relax and express yourself. The best bit is you can enjoy it at any age and in any place. You can even do it sitting in a chair! Why not?

Put on your favourite music, find your rhythm and dance yourself to fitness! You don't have to be John Travolta or Margot Fonteyn. Just let go of your inhibitions and bust some moves. Try stepping in all directions and using your whole body in any way that feels comfortable for you.

54 Trish Formby

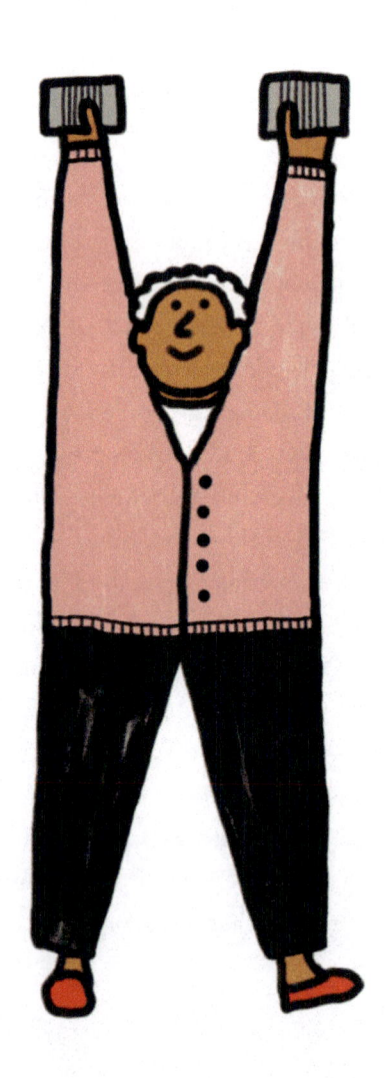

Muscling In (Arms)

As we get older, we lose muscle mass so it's really important we load up our muscles on a regular basis. Start with 'body' weight exercises, like squats or push-ups against the wall (*See* **It's a Pushover**) and slowly progress to add in light weights, like bicep curls.

You don't need a dumbbell or any kind of fancy gym kit. Just use a can of beans, a bottle of water or anything around the house that suits you. Hold the chosen 'weight' down by your side with your palm facing forward. Bend your elbow up to 90 degrees and lower. Repeat 10-15 times and then do the same with the other side or even both at the same time.

We start to lose muscle in our 30s and 40s and this deterioration accelerates as we get older and during menopause (that includes you boys!). We can lose up to a whole eight per cent of muscle mass every decade. If we lived to 200, we'd be skin and bone. The good news is that by adding weight-bearing and strength exercises to our routine – as well as making sure we have a little protein in our diet – we can slow down the loss of muscle mass. It's never too late to start! Doing weight-bearing exercises can also help with bone density loss, meaning fewer age-related fractures.

Trish Formby

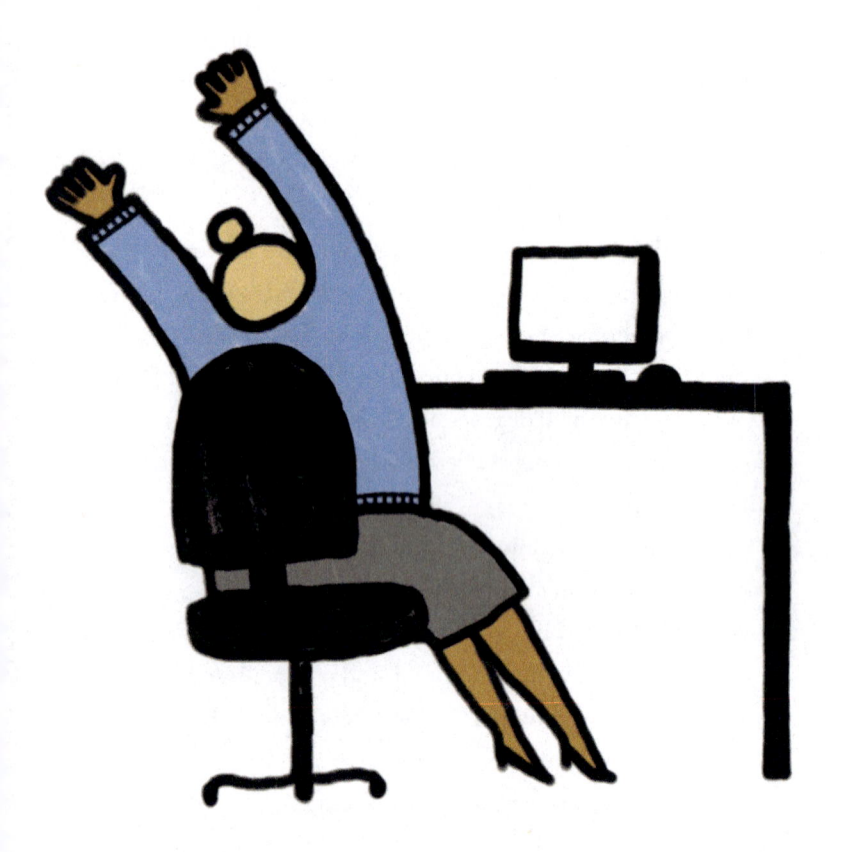

Side Hustle (Back)

'Side-bending' is a great way to mobilise your back, the gentler option if you are wary of bending backwards. It's a good general exercise to carry out after any number of activities or tasks: working a long spell at your desk, a car journey, heavy gardening, just getting up in the morning …

Stand with your feet slightly apart. Raise your right arm upwards over your head and stretch towards the left. Swap arms and repeat the other way. You can also lean your back against a wall if that feels more secure.

If your shoulders quarrel about your arms going above your head, try leaning with your arms crossed over your chest or place your hands on your head. For a quick fix when sitting at work, reach upwards and try side-bending from your chair.

If your back grouches while standing, you can try lying on the floor, facing upwards, with your arms stretched out behind your head. Make one arm longer by lengthening through your spine and then repeat with the other arm. For an added stretch, try lengthening the leg on the other side from the outstretched arm.

58 Trish Formby

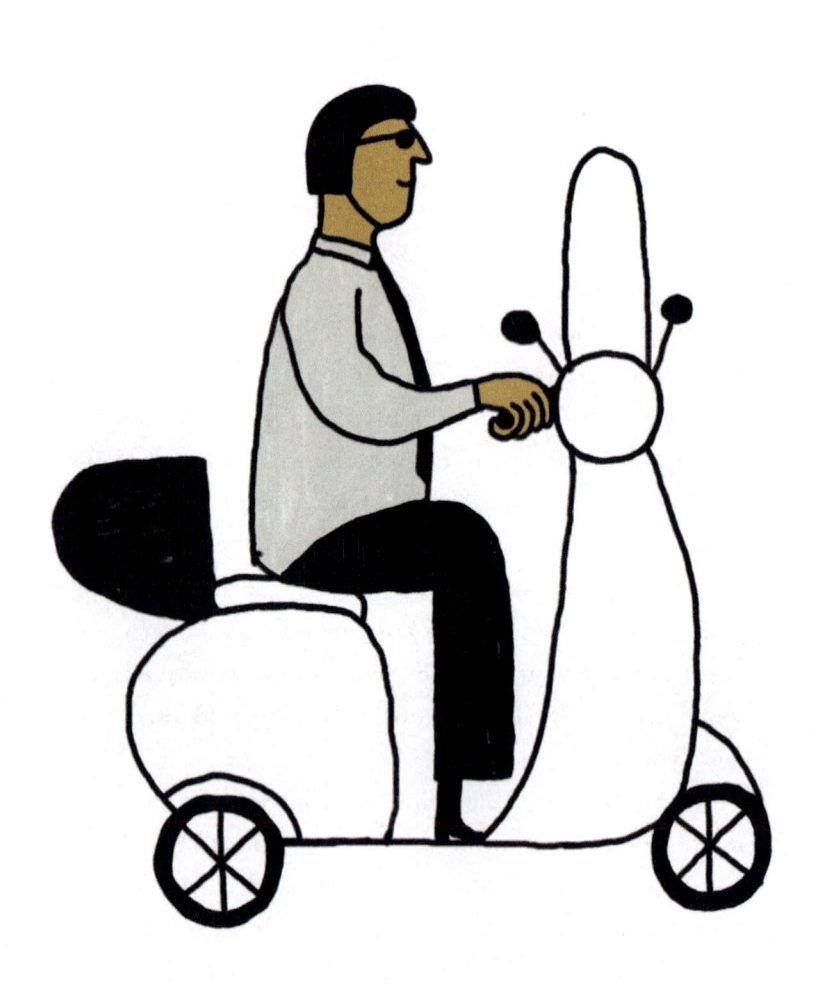

The Thin End of the Wedge (Back, Thighs)

Motorists often experience back pain. The longer the drive, the greater the pain. This can be caused, in part, by tightness in the hamstrings or the muscles at the back of the thigh. It can also be the result of sitting bolt upright and fatiguing the muscles supporting the spine.

One way to alleviate this is to use a 'wedge cushion'. Usually made of foam, the cushion is higher at the back and slopes down toward the front. This brings the hips higher than the knees helping to position the pelvis and taking some of the strain off the hamstring muscles. As with sitting for work, it is really important to take regular breaks from driving, get out of the car and go for a short walk… maybe even try some of these exercises like the **Side Hustle** or the **Twist in the Tail**!

60 Trish Formby

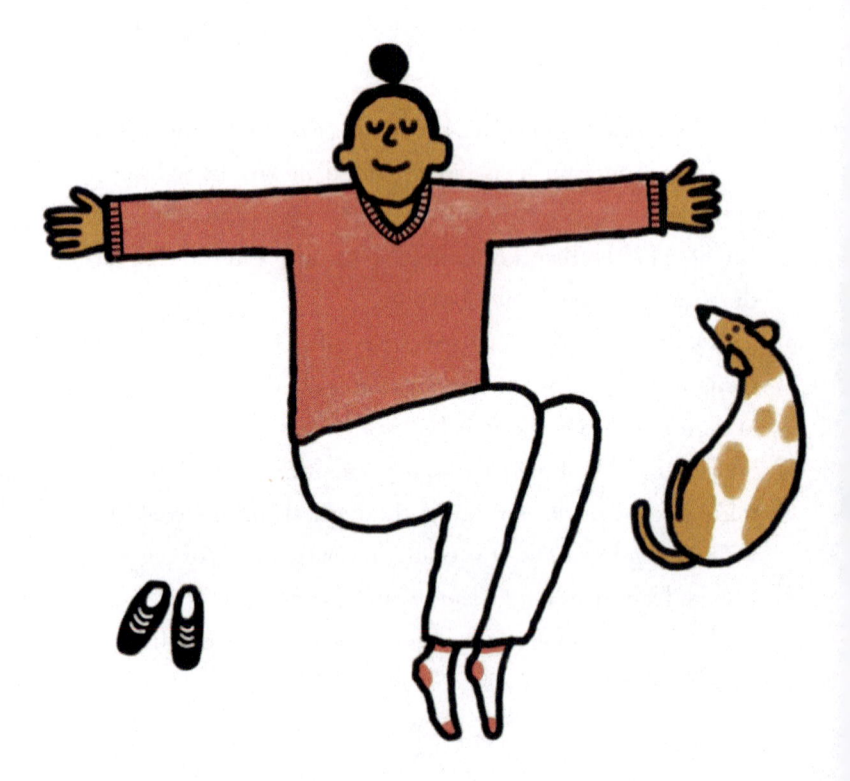

Twist in the Tail (Trunk Rotation)

Trunk rotation is an important movement for most activities from walking through to the more active sports. In most sports, we need rotation to generate power for throwing or kicking, but it's also an excellent way to mobilise your spine when you're not on the field of play.

Here's a way of doing that without leaving the home. Lie on the floor with your knees bent, feet flat and your arms in a 'stop sign' position (like a policeman stopping traffic with both arms) or stretched out (like a fallen scarecrow) to give you stability. If your shoulders complain, it's fine to place your arms down by your side.

Now roll your knees to one side as far as feels comfortable. Then roll the other way. Keep rolling side to side and then finish by bringing your knees back to the centre. Now draw your knees toward your chest, breathe deeply, exhale and stretch your legs out.

You can vary your position by crossing one knee over the other and then rolling the knees from side to side. Again, finish by bringing your knees to your chest. This stretches out the gluteals as well. Two for one!

62 Trish Formby

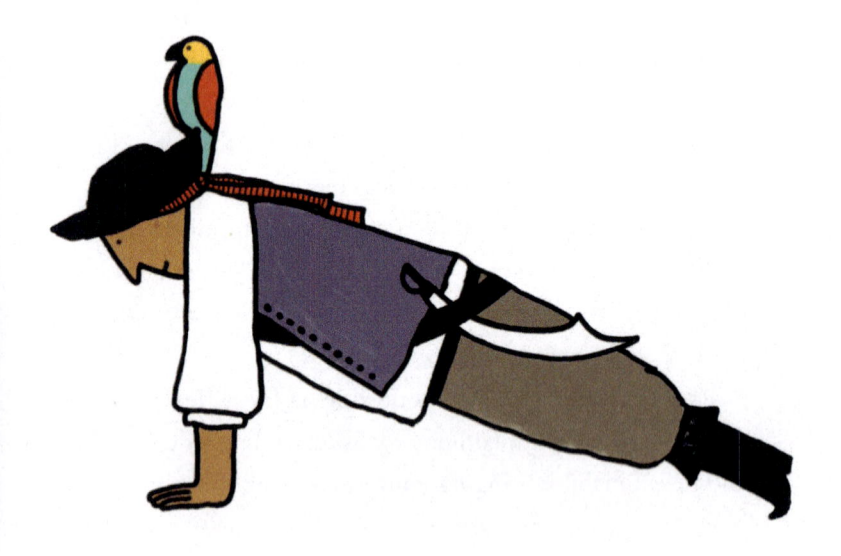

Walk the Plank (Core, Shoulders)

Planks are often performed for the core, but they are excellent for shoulder stability too as they stimulate the muscles around the shoulder blade and the deep shoulder muscles.

You don't have to perform a full hard-core plank on the floor. There are easier ways to start if you are new to them. Start by placing your hands on the edge of a table or a wall and move your feet away so you are leaning forward. Start with your elbows straight but not locked and hold the position. Now rock your weight from side to side a few times and then try rolling your weight forward and back again.

For a greater challenge, try the plank on the floor. Start by kneeling on all fours with your shoulders directly over your wrists. Extend your legs out so you are on your toes, creating a line from your head all the way down to your toes. Hold the position and then try rocking side to side and forward and back as before.

> Shoulder blade stability is essential for overhead throwing and racquet sports because it helps to optimise the function of the bigger muscles around the shoulder by providing a nice stable base for the deeper rotator cuff muscles.

64 Trish Formby

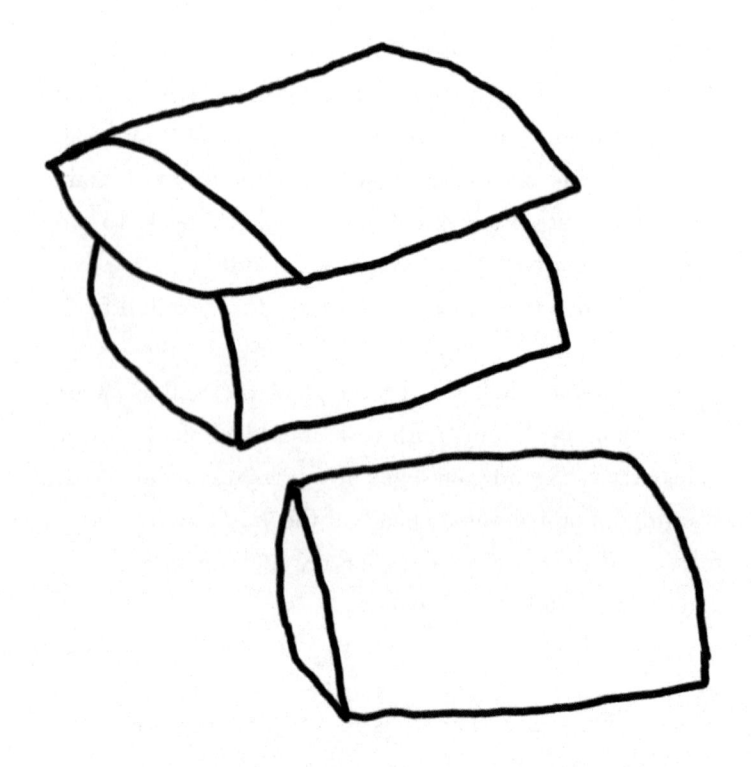

Would You Like Ice with That? (Injury)

If you have a minor acute injury, like a mild sprain or inflammation, ice can be a great way to help minimise swelling, reduce inflammation and modulate pain.

It does this by reducing blood flow through the area and so minimising the damage. It is important to do this within roughly the first 24-48 hours of sustaining the injury, and for up to 15 minutes at a time.

If the injured part is swollen, don't forget to elevate the limb above the heart. Never place ice directly on the skin. Wrap in a wet tea towel and keep checking the skin to make sure that you do not cause a painful ice burn.

> Follow the RICE protocol: Relative rest of the injured part, Ice, Compression and Elevation. You should follow this for the first 24-48 hours, depending on pain and the extent of the injury, then begin mobilising gently unless specifically advised not to.

Trish Formby

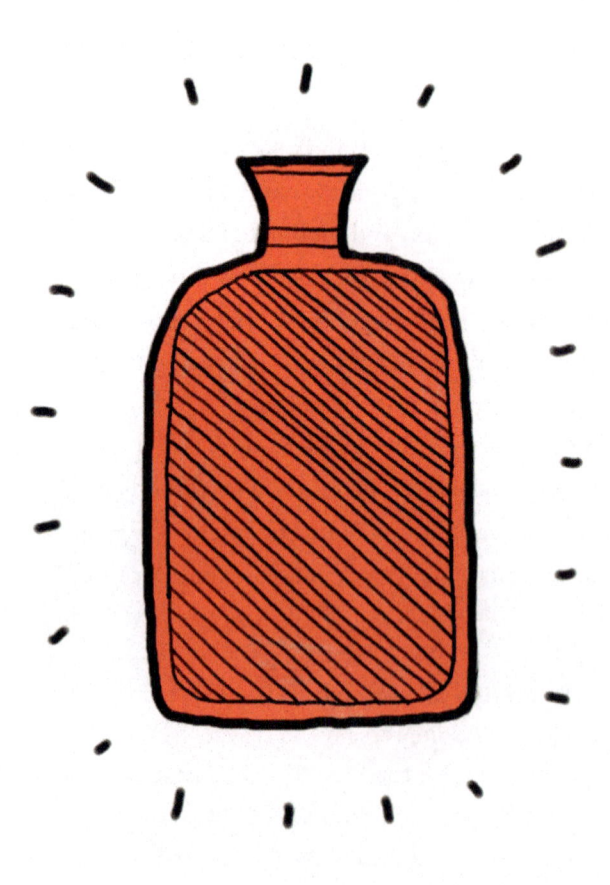

Feel The Heat (Injury)

If you suffer from stiffness or non-inflammatory pain of the muscles or joints, you might benefit from applying some heat from time to time. Heat opens up the blood vessels and stimulates better blood flow, helping to alleviate pain from muscle tightness – and promoting relaxation which also helps the pain. Try this in conjunction with **Take a Breather** with the heat across your shoulders.

A simple hot water bottle is great, but wheat and lavender bags provide a moist heat and you get the feel of it penetrating a little deeper. Whatever you use, apply it to the area you want to warm for up to 20 minutes and make sure you are in a nice, relaxed position. Just be careful that it's not too hot and keep checking the skin to make sure you don't burn yourself!

Trish Formby

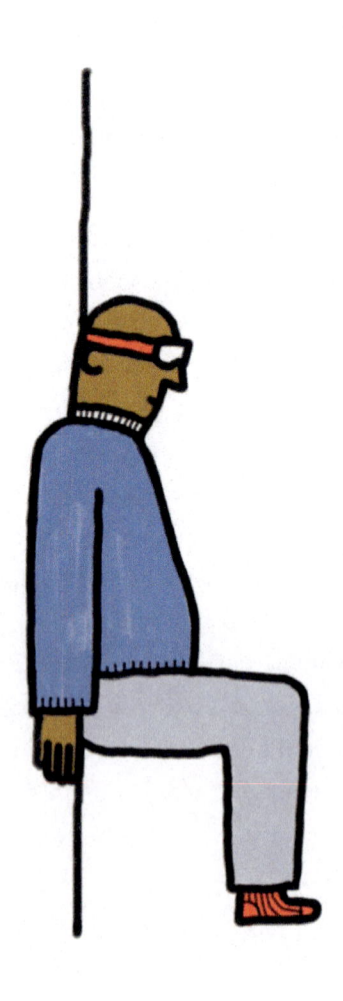

Ski Lifts & Ski Slopes (General)

Most people who go on a ski holiday don't even think about preparing for it. Big mistake. Check this out for a fact – more ski injuries happen on the last run of the last day of skiing than at any other time of the trip. That's down to the fatigue. You can avoid this, ideally for six weeks before you go, by spending just a few minutes a day doing this exercise. Stronger for it, you will reduce the chance of injuring yourself – and enjoy your skiing all the more by being fitter for the challenge.

Find a wall or door that is nice and smooth. Stand with your back to the wall and your feet about two feet away with the toes pointing forward. Now slide down the wall into a sitting position and slide back up again. Repeat 10 to15 times and then stay in the seated position and move up and down by a few inches.

Once you have mastered this, stay in the seated position, go to the next level, rise onto your toes and back down again, 10 to 15 times. Finally, cross your arms out in front of you and try rotating your trunk left and right.

Of course, it's not only the skiers who can benefit from this exercise. It's great for the quads, the gluteals, the calves and your trunk – rain, sun or snow.

70 Trish Formby

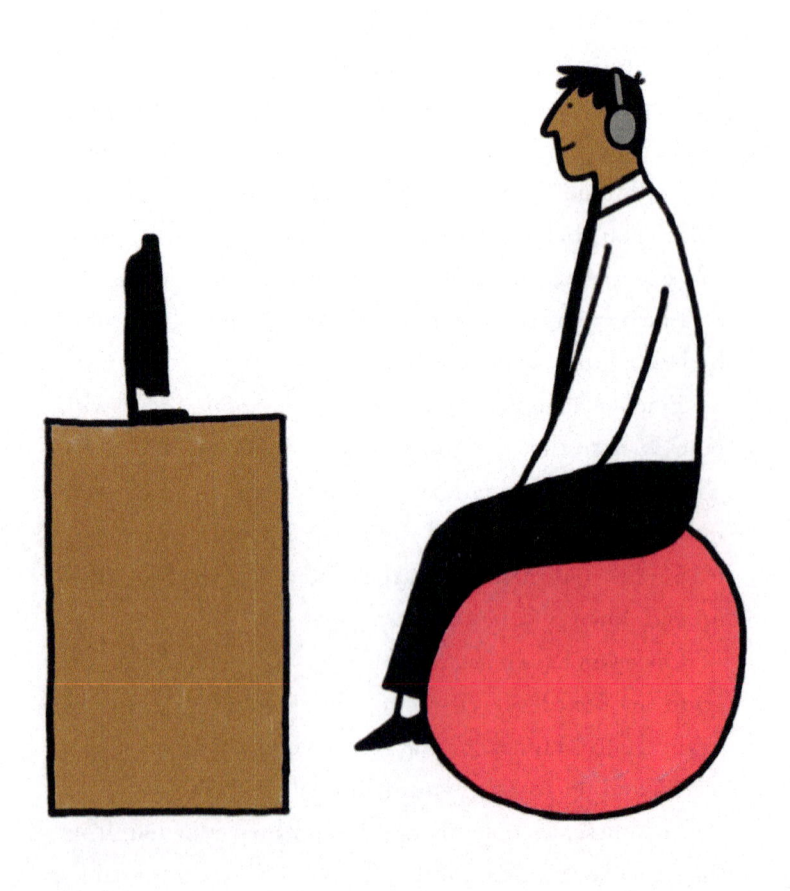

Sitting Pretty (Sitting Posture)

Many of us spend a great deal of time sitting for work. If you are a desk-jockey, try to do it so that your feet are flat, your hips are slightly higher than your knees and your head, shoulders and hips are all lined up vertically. Try not to tense or brace with your muscles, and maintain a centred position.

A good approach is to imagine lengthening through your spine and the back of your head and neck, widen the shoulders and keep them stacked over your hips. Ideally, set yourself up and then adjust your chair, if you can, to support you in your optimal position rather than trying to contort yourself to the chair.

People often think that sitting on a ball will make them sit properly but it's just as easy to slouch whilst sitting on a ball as it is in a chair. and it can be tiring if you are not used to it. However, sitting on a ball can encourage more movement whilst sitting and it's the perfect platform for exercises such as pelvic tilts or even gentle bouncing with the added benefit of challenging our balance a little more and that's a good thing.

> Many people spend up to nine hours sitting a day! Sitting for that long can slow the metabolism, reduce blood flow and cause stiffness in the hips and upper back. Sitting with better posture will also help your breathing and, if you give presentations, will help with projecting your voice and make you look more confident. That goes for standing too.

Trish Formby

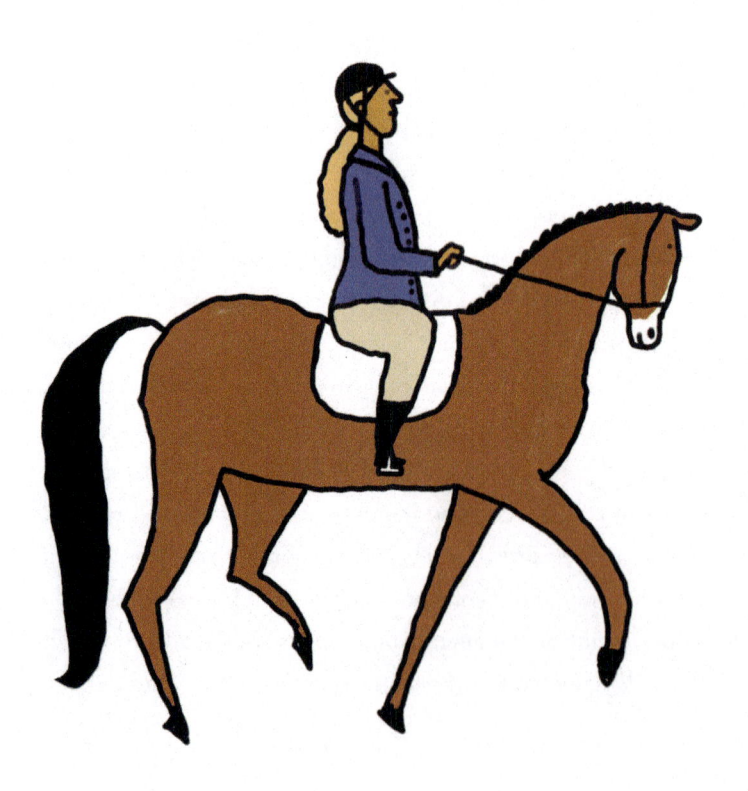

Horsing Around (Hamstrings)

The hamstrings fulfil a multi-purpose function, similar to the adductors. They play a role in bending the knee, adducting the leg, stabilising the pelvis and controlling the extension of the knee during sprinting and running.

Critically, the hamstrings also act like brakes to slow the leg down just before we strike the ground with our foot. The faster we move and, more crucially, the longer the stride that we take, the more the hamstrings have to absorb the braking forces. If I had a pound for every time a middle-aged man has limped into clinic having torn his hamstring at the school sports day… and of course, they were always just about to break the tape before disaster struck!

This little exercise is one I used to give to sprinters and footballers, but it's a good one for all of us.

Stand on one leg, nice and tall, and bend your hip and knee to 90 degrees. Pull your foot upward. Now extend your leg straight out in front of you keeping your toes up. Then, keeping the knee straight lower down to the floor, bring the knee up again to your starting point. Think one-legged cycling action! Do ten repetitions and each time, hold the start position with your hip and knee at 90 degrees.

Once you can balance and control the exercise, speed up so that each flick is fast, but always hold between each repetition. You can also add light weights around the ankle.

Please give this one to all Dads a few weeks ahead of school Sports Day!

Trish Formby

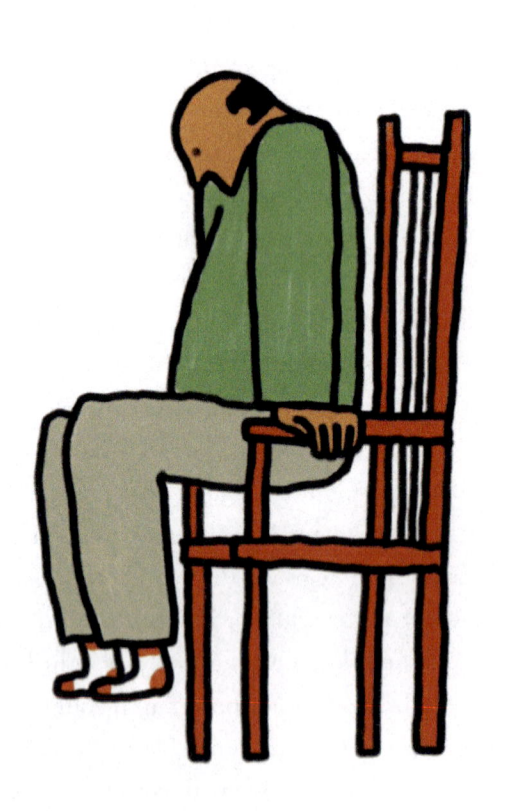

We Have Lift-Off (Shoulders, Arms)

This exercise helps with shoulder stability and firms up the triceps, the muscles at the back of the upper arms, otherwise known as 'bingo wings' when they have lost their firmness!

If you have armrests place your hands on them, level with your hips, and widen your shoulders. Press down and lift your bottom from the chair 10 to 15 times. You can keep your feet on the ground but try not to push too hard through your legs. As you get better, you can take more weight through your arms.

If you do not have armrests, place your hands down by your hips on your knuckles and press downward straightening your elbows and lifting your bottom off the chair.

76 Trish Formby

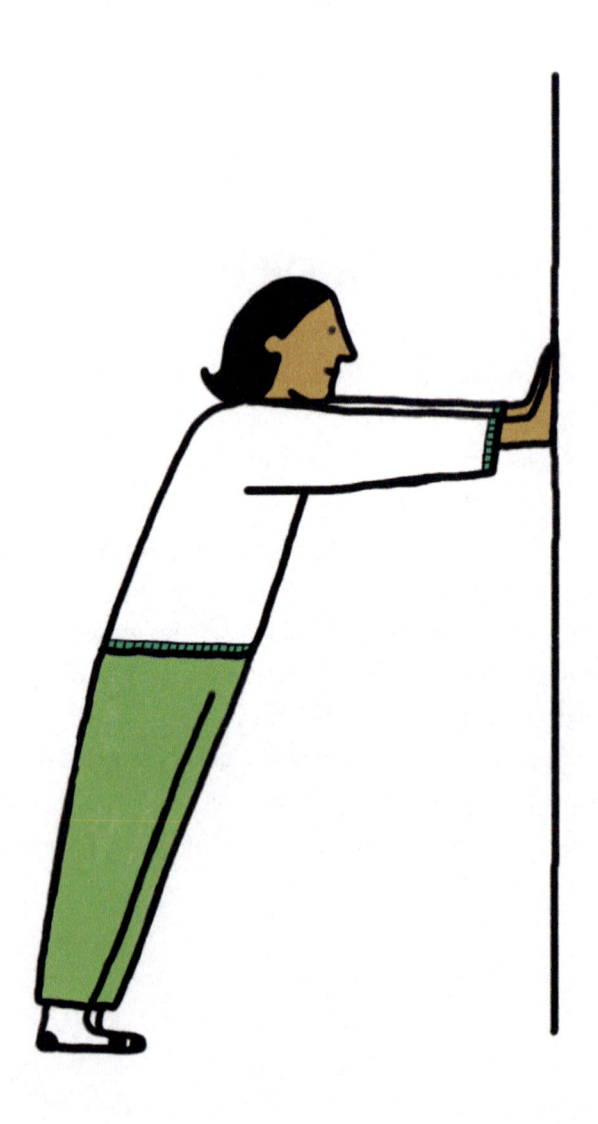

You're a Pushover (Shoulders, Arms)

Push-ups don't have to be done on the floor. Many people just don't have the strength for it, but there is another, less stressful way: do them against a wall. This exercise is still highly beneficial for the shoulders and arms, especially the triceps.

Stand a few feet away from the wall and place your hands shoulder-width apart on the wall – at shoulder height. Bend your elbows so that your forehead moves toward the wall and then straighten out again. Repeat 10 to 15 times. Build up more repetitions as you get stronger. You can increase the load by leaning on a table. Who knows? You might even become strong enough to hit the floor and try the classic push-up.

Trish Formby

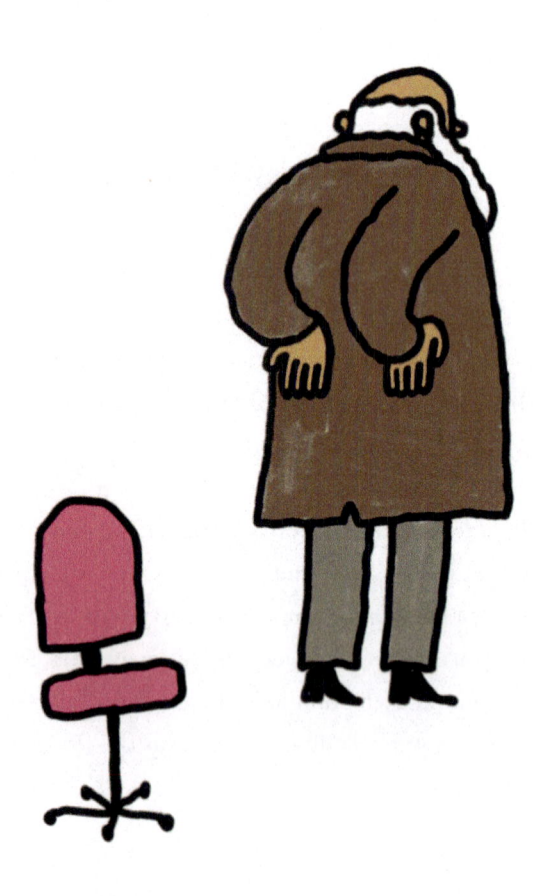

Hip & Bendy (Hip)

Sitting at a desk all day can make your back, neck and hips feel really stiff and generally make you a little chair shaped by the end of the day.

Try stretching out at the end of your bed or even better, at the top of the stairs! Sit on the landing at the top, then place both feet on the second or third step. Bring your right knee up to the chest and roll back into a lying position keeping the left foot on the stair.

If you can, press the left heel down and into the upright of the step. You should feel a stretch across the front of your hip. If there are no stairs available, you can also do this one at the end of your bed. There's always something or somewhere in the home!

Fun fact: Apparently the first person to add wheels to their chair thus creating the first 'office chair' was Charles Darwin in the 1800's. He did this so he could whizz about to his many desks so he was probably also the first person to experience back pain from prolonged sitting. We now use wheels for office Olympic races, way more fun

80   Trish Formby

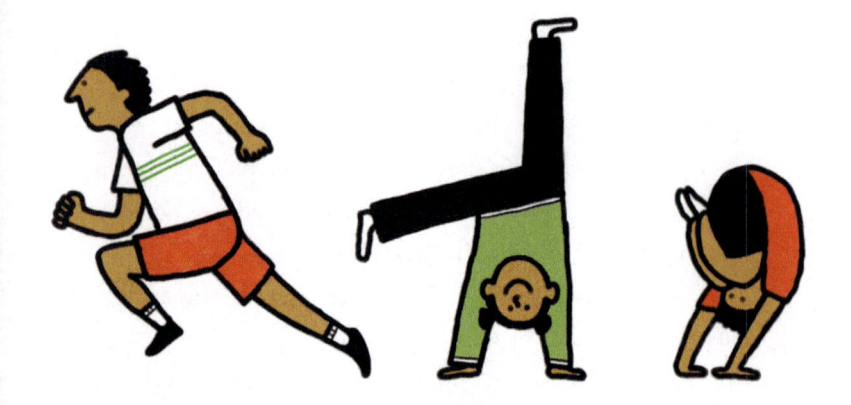

Child's Play (Whole Body)

Have you ever noticed the amazing posture and flexibility of children? When kids engage in free play they move and stretch in all directions and don't follow the patterns we do when we get older. Patterns of movement only start once we engage in more formal sports training and prolonged sitting in lessons.

Consequently, we develop 'asymmetries' in our mobility, and stiffness, which we don't necessarily notice until much later. These can worsen as patterns become more ingrained.

So, make like a kid now and then! Run around in circles, try rolling, jumping, bending, crawling and skipping or play a game, play with a pet or better still, play with a kid! As an added benefit you might just feel like a kid again.

> Did you know that hobby horsing is a thing? Yes, really. It started in Finland but has since been taken up in Sweden, Germany and the UK. Hobby horsing is a sport in which fully grown adults perform the competitive routines of equestrian horse jumping on a hobby horse. There is even a world championship which, in 2022, attracted over 1,500 competitors. Guaranteed to bring a smile to your face (See **Go on Give us a Smile**) it will get you fit – and it's way cheaper than buying a horse.

82   Trish Formby

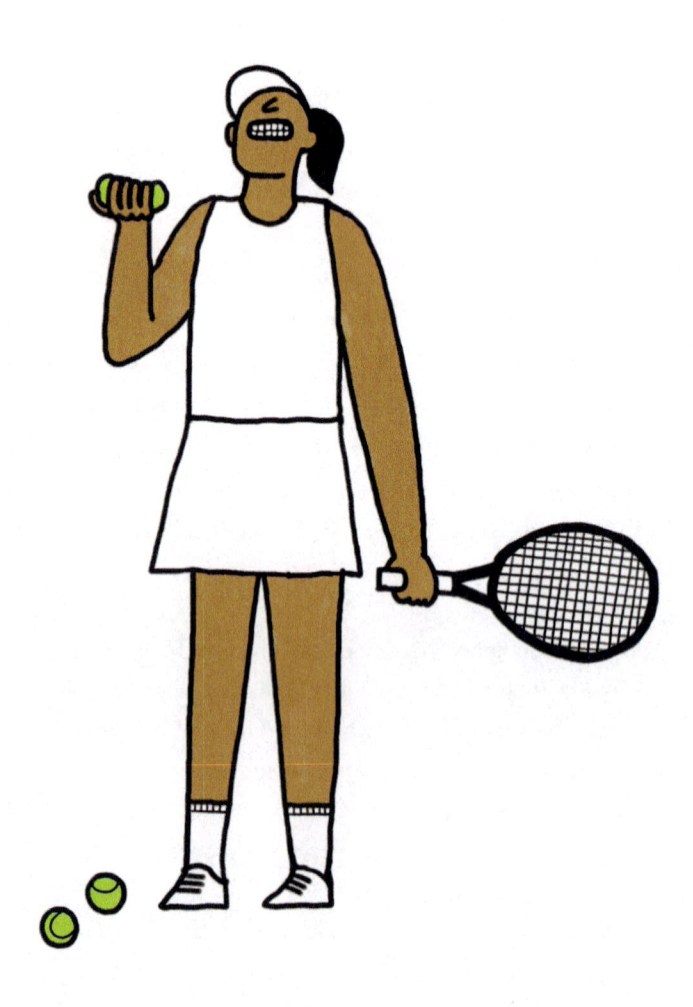

Get a Grip (Hand, Wrist)

Grip strength is a really good indicator of overall strength and health. Typically, grip strength will peak in midlife and decline with age. Studies have shown that reduced grip strength can be a good predictor of cardiac health and longevity.

Although doing exercises to maintain grip strength will not prolong life, it is still important for many daily functions such as carrying things, opening jars and picking things up.

Hold a filled water bottle and rest your forearm on a table or desk. With the palm facing upwards, flex your wrist toward your forearm and repeat 10 to 15 times. Then do the same with the palm facing downwards, extending the wrist.

Squeezing a tennis ball is also a good wrist strengthener with the bonus of being a fantastic stress-buster… if you're watching the news or having an awkward conversation.

84 Trish Formby

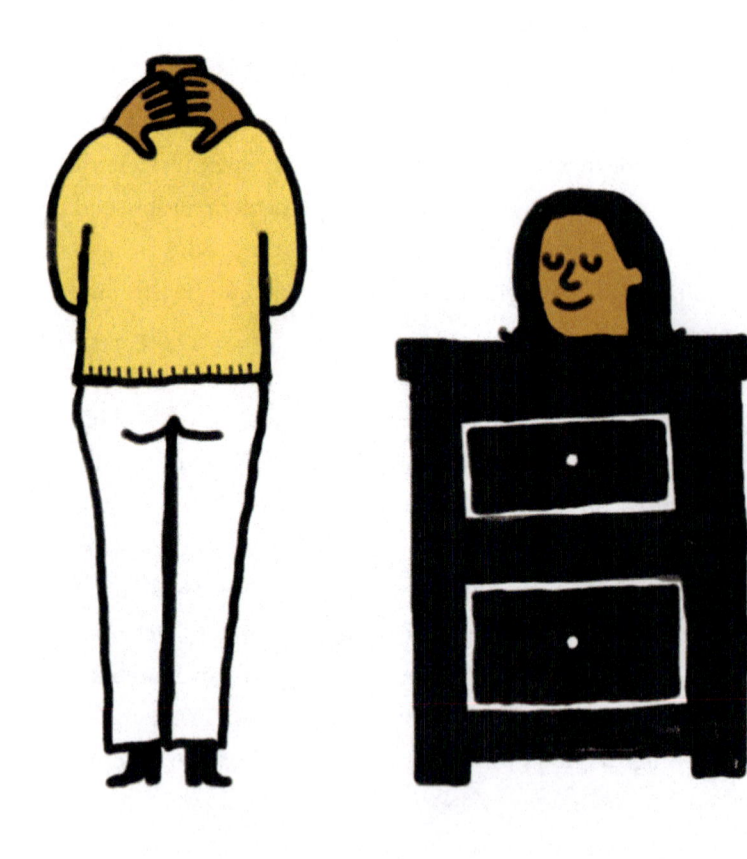

Where's Your Head At? (Neck)

Your head position helps dictate the position of the rest of your body, influencing vision, balance, hearing, swallowing and changing direction.

When the head and neck are in a neutral position, the weight of the head is distributed evenly across the muscles of the neck. This is best for prolonged positions as it minimises stress through the muscles and the joints of the spine.

To help achieve this position, line up your ear lobes over your shoulders and lengthen the back of the neck. Slightly drop the chin whilst maintaining a central position of the head on the shoulders and picture a piece of string from the crown of your head gently pulling you taller.

> Your head weighs around 4.5 to 5kg. That's really heavy! No wonder our neck muscles get tired after a long day at a screen. If you are looking down, the strain of the head on the neck increases to around 8kg at 15 degrees and 10kg at 30 degrees. Ten kilos is the weight of a microwave. That's a hefty load for a neck to bear!

86   Trish Formby

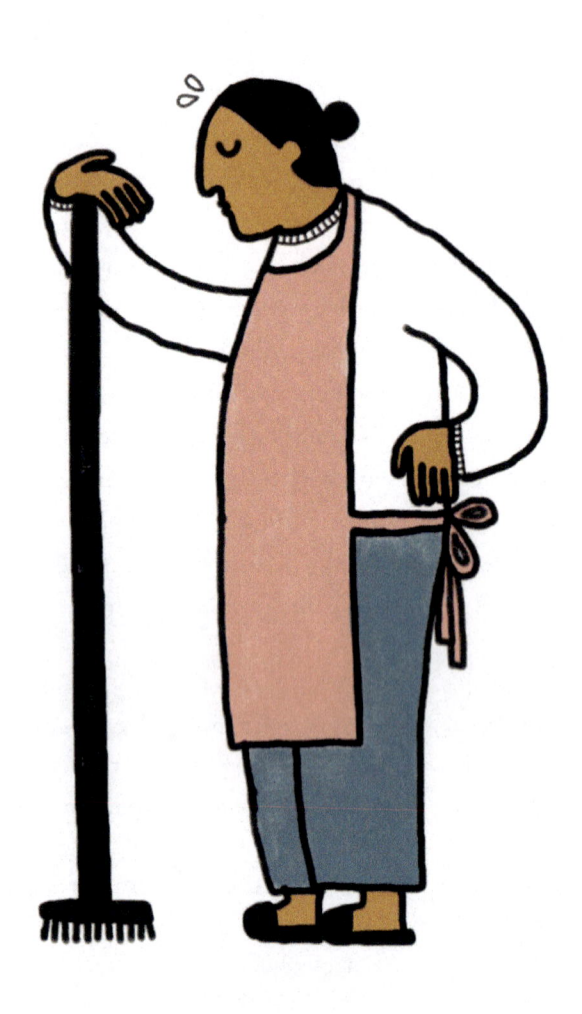

Housework (Whole Body – and some)

It's not just sport that can cause pain and injuries. Household chores such as vigorous vacuuming, scrubbing, sweeping and ironing are a common cause of repetitive strain injuries. The body areas most likely to suffer repetitive strain are the wrists, elbows and shoulders. Often, this will occur after a good spring-clean or clearing up after a particularly good party!

Prolonged or repetitive overhead tasks are also a major cause of shoulder pain, so invest in a good step stool to work at around shoulder height where possible or, even better, somewhere between hip and shoulder.

Make sure you take regular breaks and keep varying the tasks and your body position. For example, if you have been vacuuming, try following up with something a bit less demanding that uses a completely different position. If you have been kneeling for a task, then make the next job a standing one or, better still, try some of the stretches in this book to break up your work.

> The number one cause of injuries in our home are slips, trips and falls from wet floors, loose rugs and clutter. Around 2.7 million people end up in A&E every year after injuring themselves at home. Make sure you have plenty of space around you before you clean, get help moving heavy furniture, wear proper supportive shoes and use tape to hold rugs if necessary.

88 Trish Formby

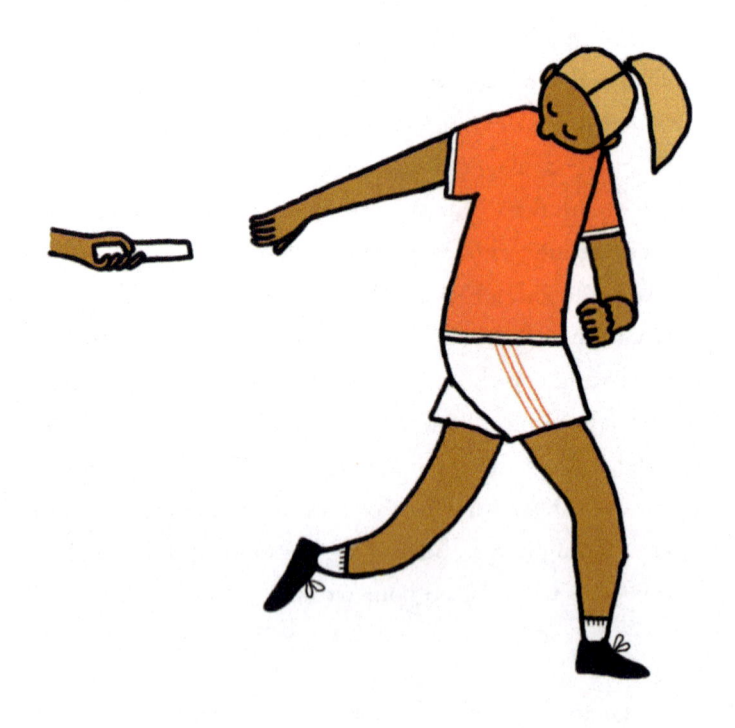

Pass the Baton (Forearms, Elbows)

If you spend a lot of time at a keyboard or you have been doing a task that involves gripping, you might find that you get stiff in your forearms and sore on your outer elbows (the 'lateral' elbow). If this gets worse, it can develop into something misleadingly called 'tennis elbow'. Most people with tennis elbow don't even play tennis! To alleviate the tension and prevent elbow pain, try this stretch.

Place your thumb across your palm to the base of your little finger and make a fist over it. Then flex your fist toward your wrist. Stretch your arm out behind you with your fist facing upwards. It's similar to the position that relay runners use to receive the baton in a relay race. You should feel a good stretch in your forearm. Take the arm off the stretch by bending your elbow and then extend again. Repeat 4 to 5 times on both arms (separately) every hour or so. Also, make sure you mobilise your upper back and neck (*See* **Don't Get the Hump, Bow & Arrow**)

> Although up to 50 per cent of tennis players will experience elbow pain during their career, only 2 to 3 per cent of all lateral elbow pain cases are actually caused by tennis.

Trish Formby

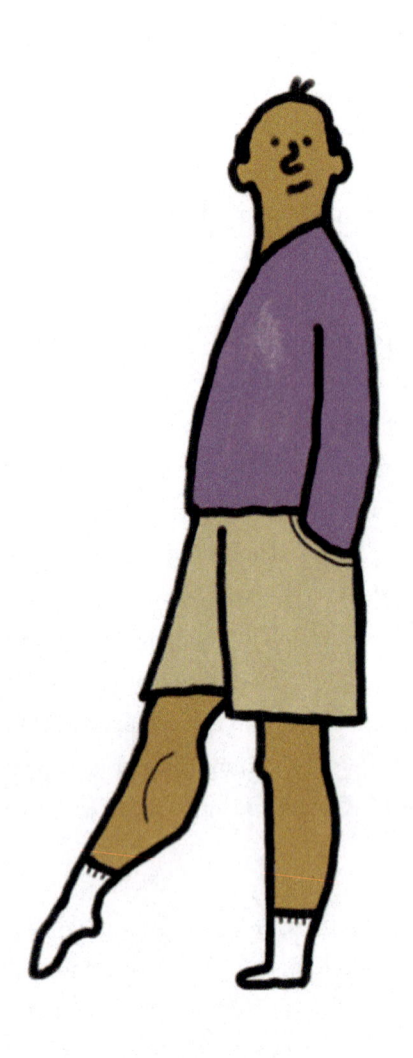

The Ankle Angle (Ankle & More!)

People often suffer from stiffness in the ankles, particularly when enacting what is known clinically as 'dorsi-flexion'. In layman's terms, this means the action of pulling your foot upwards toward your leg. This will also occur in a weight-bearing position when lunging forward and your knee goes over your toes. Reduced range in 'dorsi-flexion' is often the result of old ankle injuries, sprains, Achilles tendinopathy, shortness in the calf muscles or bone spurs.

Typically, we need about 10 to 25 degrees of dorsiflexion for normal daily activity (it varies depending on which studies you read!) In short, we need it for walking, lunging, hill-walking, running and so on. A lack of mobility in this regard can have an unwelcome domino effect, leading to stress and strain in other areas.

This stretch is a simple way to improve and maintain ankle mobility. Place the big toe of your foot against a wall with the foot pointing straight forward and the heel grounded. Now bend your knee over your middle toe toward the wall. Once you are touching the wall with your knee, slide the foot away from the wall until you feel a stretch at the back of the ankle. Make sure you keep that heel on the floor! Hold this position for around 30 seconds.

To double-down on improving this range do the calf raises (*See* **All Rise**) and the bent knee calf raises (*See* **Bent Knee Calf Raise**) These are more suitable for tendinopathies rather than stretching.

92 Trish Formby

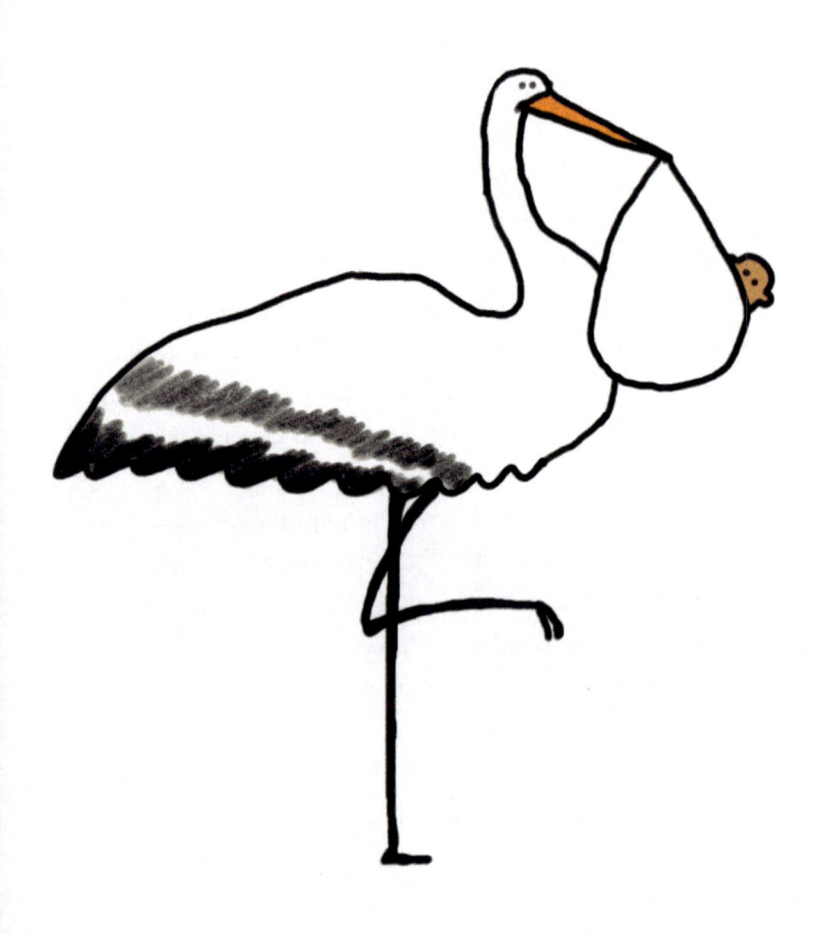

Stand like a Stork (Legs)

One for the experts! Sit on a bench or chair with the hips slightly higher than the knees. Now take your left foot off the ground and move from sitting to standing on your right leg. Try to keep your kneecap over your middle toe. Repeat 10 times and then try the other leg.

If you are struggling to do the exercise, sit sideways on a sturdy dining room chair with the back of it on your right side. Place your right hand on the back of the chair, lift your right foot off the ground and assist yourself to stand on the left leg. The added benefit of this modification is that you work your triceps too! Repeat 10 times and then sit facing the opposite way to do the other leg.

94   Trish Formby

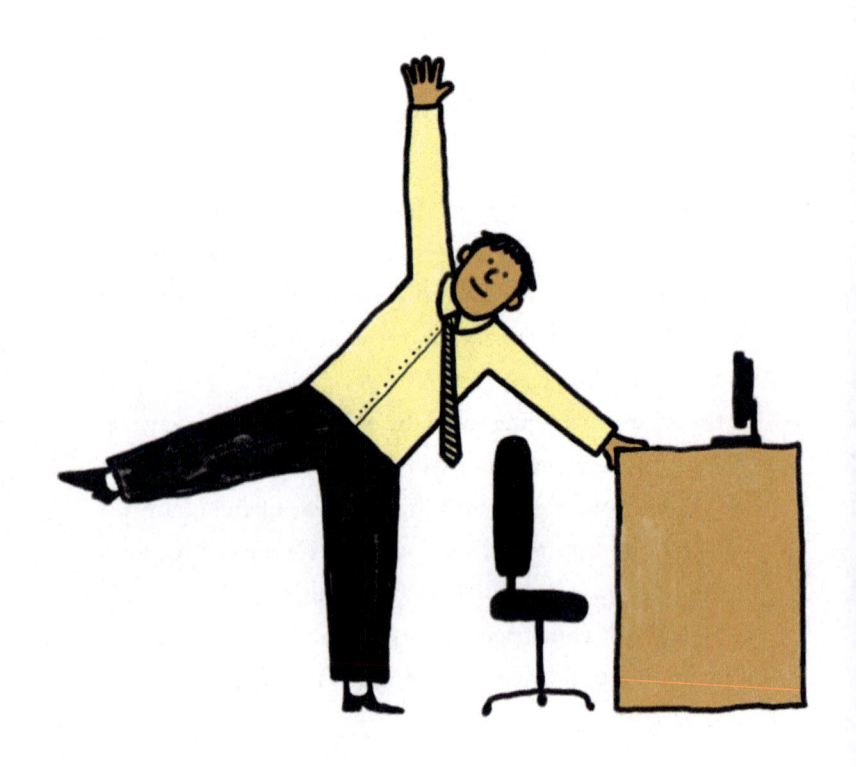

Side Plank (Shoulders, Glutes)

Side planks using your desk, table or kitchen surfaces are excellent for your shoulder stability – and you get to add in a little gluteal work at the same time. You can use a wall too.

Stand side-on to your support and place your right hand on the edge of the surface. Move your feet a little away from your desk until your body is inclined at an angle to the floor and you are supported by your arm. Make your arm longer and lengthen through your body as far as you can. Now extend your left arm out to the side. Hold this position for 30 seconds and then repeat on the other side.

For a tougher challenge, try lifting the outer leg straight out to the side so you make a 'star' shape with your body.

Why not throw in a side bend at the end? If you are resting on your right arm, try leaning your body sideways over to the right and reach over your head with your left arm.

Trish Formby

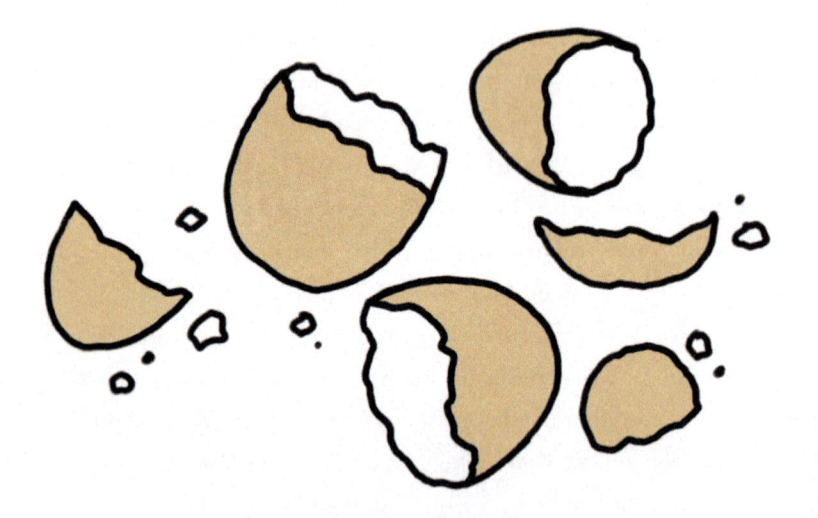

Prepare for Landing! (Balance)

… or as a pilot once said to a trainee after a particularly rough landing, 'Sonny, did we land, or did we get shot down?'

When we walk, jump, run, hop or skip we are absorbing heavy forces coming up from the ground and using our muscles to protect our joints and ligaments from the impact. Landing with stiff or rigid knees can lead to damage of the knee joint, as well as areas further up the body, especially the hips and lower back.

This little exercise helps to train the body for a nice smooth landing.

Stand on the first step of the stairs or a low stable step. Step forward onto your right leg. As you land, try to point your foot directly forward and bend your knee, keeping your kneecap over your middle toe. Land as lightly as you can, as if you were stepping on eggshells and trying not to break them. Allow your knee to bend enough to make the landing smooth.

As you get better at landing, try a little jump off the step and land on one leg but make sure you bend your knee enough as you land and then hold the position on one leg to finish (balance).

98 Trish Formby

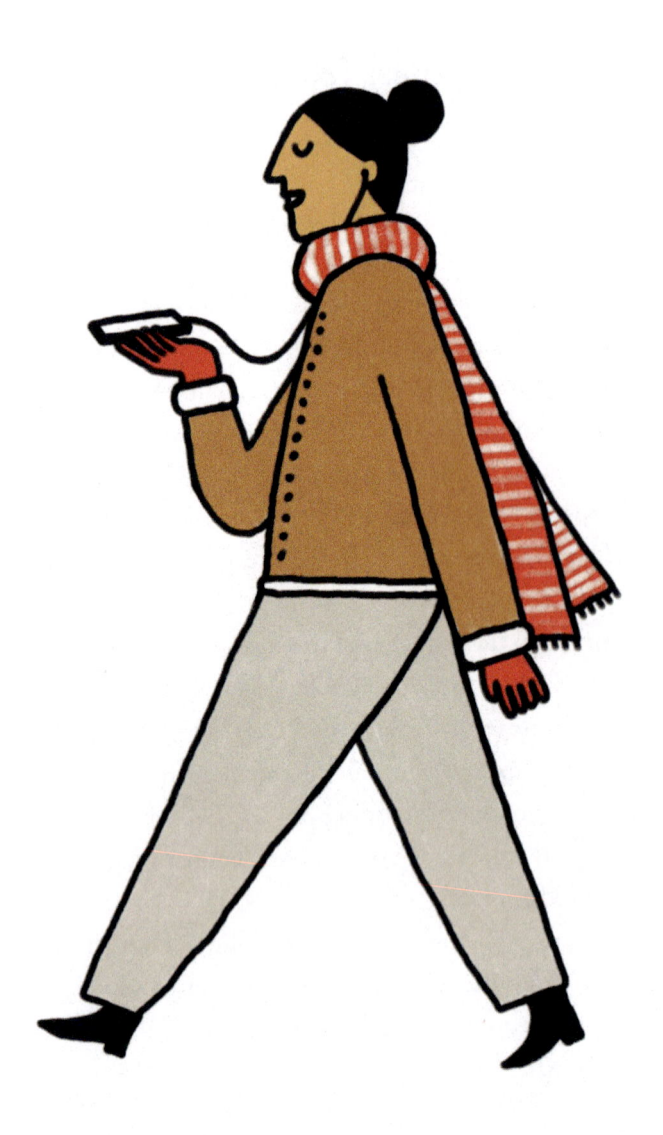

Walk and Talk (Whole Body)

If you are someone who spends a lot of time on the phone, to work colleagues, friends or family, try popping in some earbuds or headphones and go for a 'virtual' walk with them. You may find you are more receptive to their requests, demands or moans!

Walking is the easiest and most accessible exercise that most of us can do without difficulty. This everyday action stimulates circulation and promotes oxygen to the brain. The quicker the better. It is also good for bone health because it is weight-bearing and, little and often, it can help with maintaining a healthy weight.

Try walking briskly for 10 minutes daily to start and build up from there. Make sure you swing your arms and, if you have balance issues, use walking poles in both hands so that you encourage trunk rotation and natural arm swing i.e. the arms swinging in step with the opposite leg. Try walking with the same side arm and leg going forward at the same time. It feels really strange but don't do this for long! You might not be able to stop.

100 Trish Formby

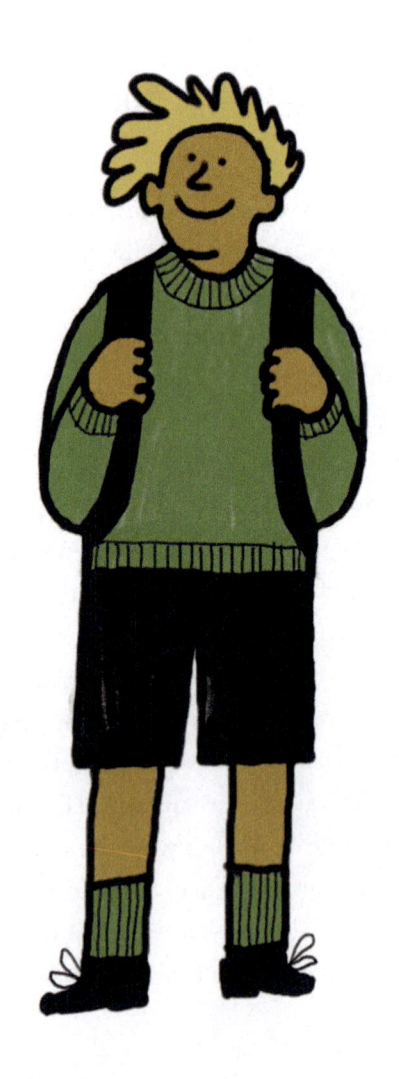

Backpacking (Back)

If you need to carry lots of items around with you during the day such as laptops and books, a good backpack is a must. If you use quite a heavy one for long periods, it is important to wear it and load it well to avoid developing poor posture, muscle imbalance and joint stress. Worn well and packed properly, a backpack offers a workout while you go about business.

Backpacks distribute the load across the shoulders so that we can maintain an upright position and walk with a natural arm swing and rotation. Loading up evenly through the spine will also help you to engage your core because the compression encourages the deep muscles around your spine and abdominals to switch on.

Choosing the right backpack is important. Depending on how much weight you are planning to carry, you may need one with wider straps so that they don't dig into your shoulders. If you are carrying more weight, a waist belt can be a great help because it takes some of the load through the hips. Make sure the straps are adjustable and use them when putting the backpack on and taking off — rather than having a wrestling match with it and half-dislocating your shoulders every time!

You might also like to use a weighted vest or backpack to add load when you are walking or doing weight-bearing exercises such as squats or calf raises. If you are planning a hiking holiday this can be a really good way to train. Start by adding light weights and slowly build up over time. Allow a good 4 to 6 weeks of training to work up to the weight you will be carrying, and you will be fit to travel!

102   Trish Formby

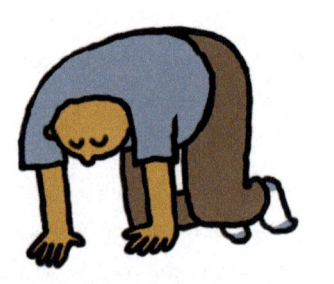

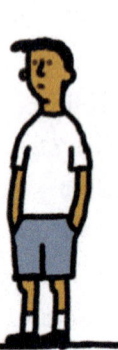

Hovercraft (Whole Body)

Kneeling on your hands and knees is a pretty good exercise in itself, creating a gentle compressive force through the hips and the shoulders and encouraging the deeper muscles around the joints to get to work.

As with our spine, we have deeper muscles around our hips and shoulders, which help to guide and control movement. When these muscles are all in balance, we establish good smooth movement in our major joints and that's important if you want them to age well.

Here's a pleasurable yoga-style routine for the set-up, similar to the pose sometimes called the cat-and-cow, and ending in a neutral spine. Find a nice space on the floor. Ideally, use a mat or floor with a softer surface. Wood or tiles are too harsh on the kneecaps. Kneel on the floor with your hands and knees shoulder-width apart. Try to make sure your hands are directly under your shoulders and your knees directly under your hips.

Now curl your back upwards and then arch downwards. Do this a few times because it feels very satisfying, then settle somewhere in the middle with a 'neutral spine' and lengthen through your neck so you are looking at the floor. From here you can rock your weight gently forward and back or side to side. Or you can try stretching one leg out behind you for more of a challenge in every way. Stretch the opposite arm out in front.

To increase the load, turn your feet under so that you are on your toes and then 'hover' your knees above the ground. Hold this position for 45 seconds and repeat three times.

Trish Formby

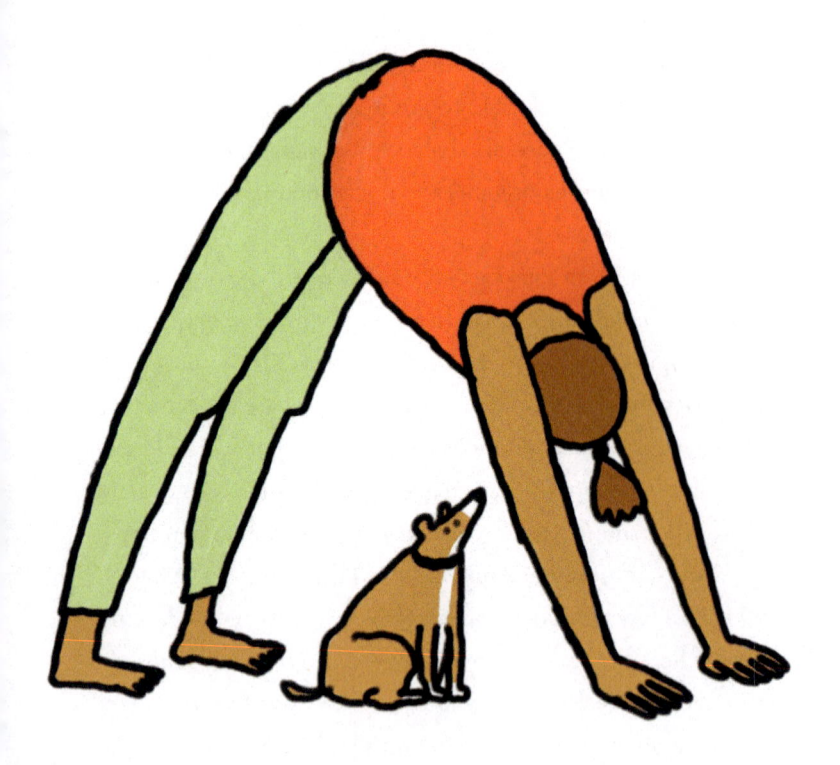

Do the Pike (Legs, Shoulders)

This is a great position to stretch out the back of the legs and the shoulders. It's commonly known in yoga as the 'downward dog' but you don't need to be a yogi or a dog to do it!

Start in a four-point kneeling position on the floor, that is, on your hands and knees with your spine in a neutral position. Rest your toes on the floor and take a nice deep breath. On the breath out, lift from your tailbone so that you straighten your knees and rise onto your toes.

Imagine that there is a belt around your hips, and you are being lifted upward. Extend as far as you feel comfortable and, once there, you can 'walk' your feet so that you alternately press your heels to the floor. Take another deep breath and lower down on the breath out. Repeat three times.

106 Trish Formby

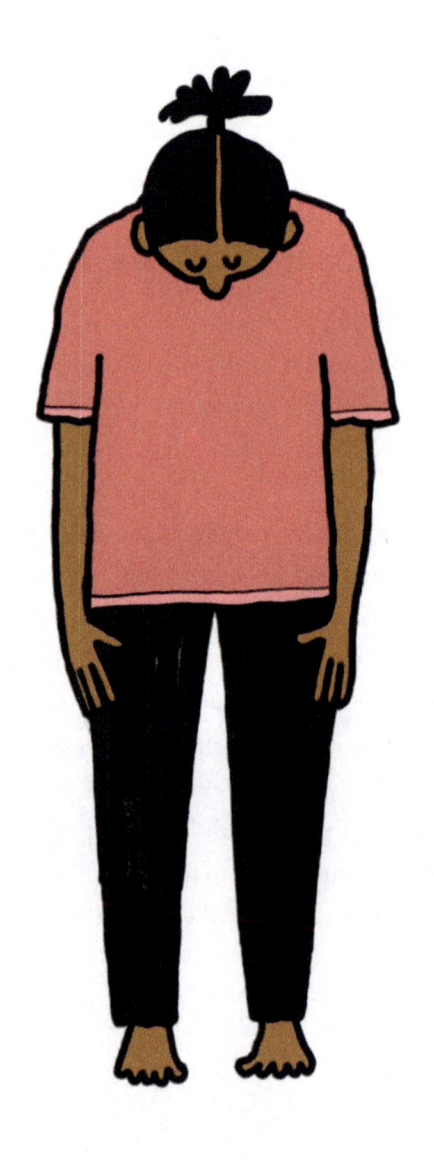

Salute Your Unsung Little Heroes (Adductors)

Poor little adductors – they work really hard every day, and we don't even appreciate, or know, that they are carrying out a whole range of functions for us!

These are the four muscles on the inside of our thighs that have a stabilising role at the pelvis and are active when we walk or stand on one leg. They also allow 'adduction' of the leg — that's the fancy term for bringing the leg across closer to our midline, as when we are kicking crossways. And that's not all. They assist the pelvic floor and the hamstrings and even help us to bend our knees. These are awesome little muscles that deserve our undying respect and gratitude!

Here's a little routine to show them some kindness. Lie on the floor on your side with your top leg resting on a chair. Now lift the bottom leg to meet the top leg without rolling off your side. You can use your arms to keep your balance but try not to push too hard. Lift and repeat 10 to 15 times then roll over to the other side and do the other leg. Alternatively, try dancing like Elvis 'The Pelvis' Presley! (*See* **Kitchen Disco**)

Trish Formby

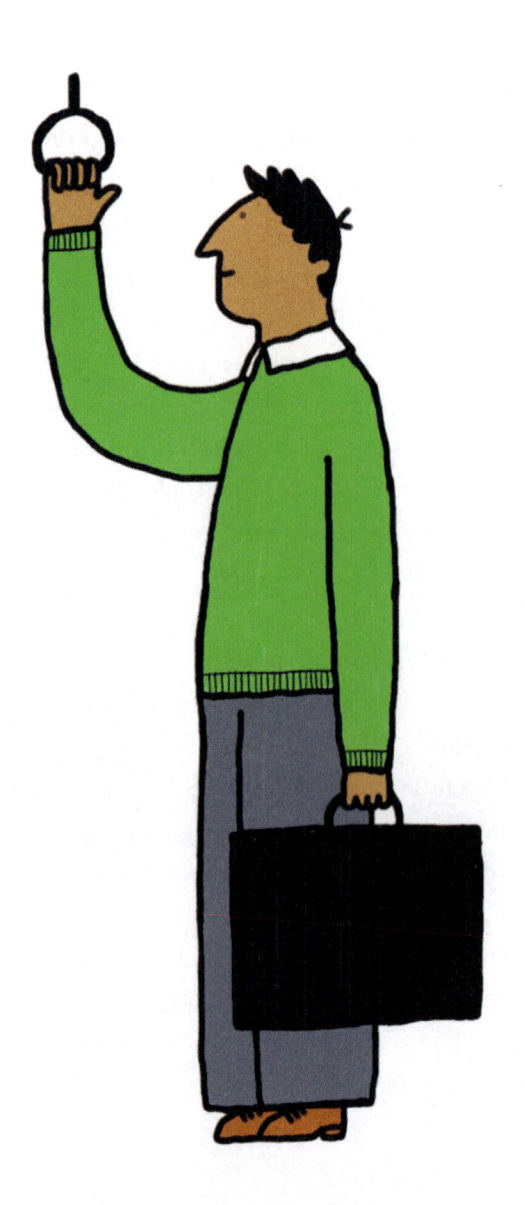

Stand and Deliver (Whole Body)

Many of us must work by spending hours sitting at a desk every day. That's the way of the modern world. Those hours can really add up and take a heavy toll on our bodies.

Standing to work is a brilliant way to improve your postural endurance — and, using up to 95 calories per hour, that's also a plus, considering you are rooted to the spot. Another bonus of standing is that it encourages more oxygen to the brain, enhancing memory, productivity, creativity and problem-solving.

If you invest in a standing desk – and I highly recommend that you do – stand with your weight evenly distributed and try to keep your neck long and your shoulders centred over your hips. You should be in a relaxed position without tension in your back. (*See* **My Work Here Is Done** for general desk set-up).

If you can't find a place around the house where you can set up a standing workplace, try standing each time you need to make a phone call or try taking meetings whilst upright. If you are a commuter on a bus or train, then give up your seat and stand instead. Win some fitness and thanks all in one! This will improve your balance in small but significant ways over time.

Standing all day can be very tiring, especially when you first start, so always have regular breaks to move and loosen up. Start with 10 to 15 minutes each hour and then increase the time as you feel able. Listen to your body! It always knows best.

Trish Formby

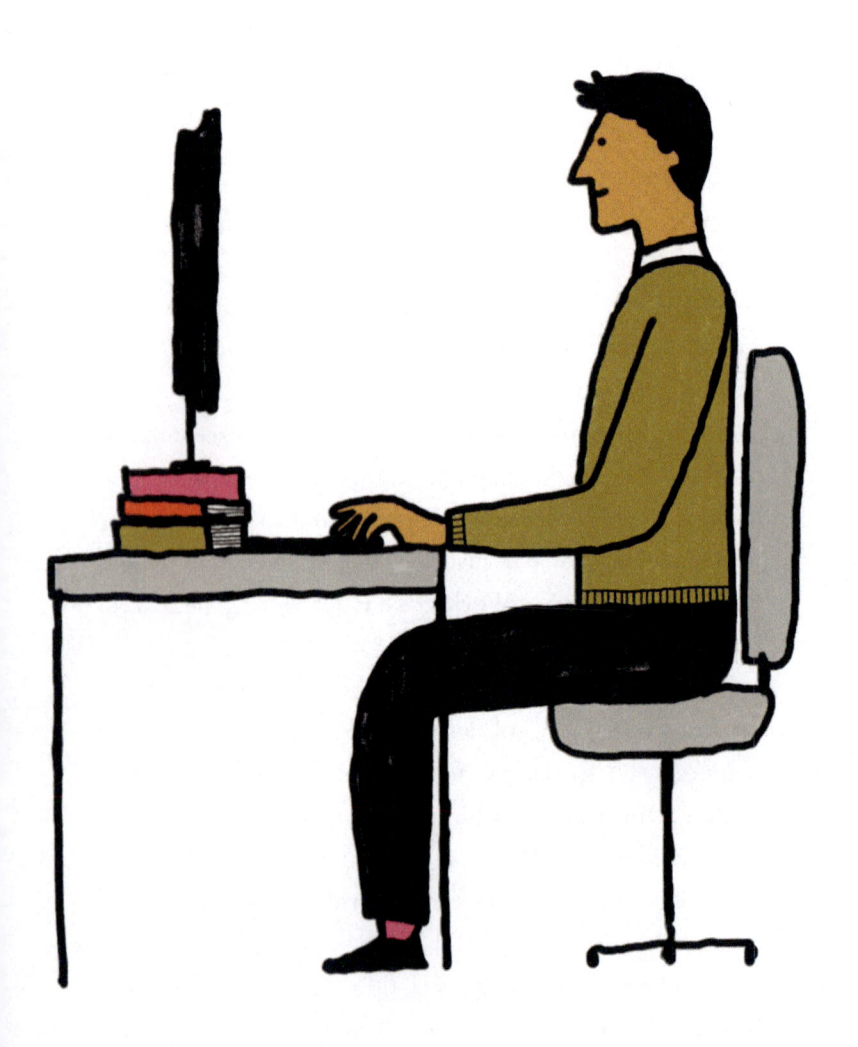

My Work Here is Done (Whole Body)

Whether working from home or in an office, whether you sit or stand, a well set-up workplace will help to alleviate the aches and pains of a long day. It's important that you set up your body position first and then adjust your equipment to help you maintain that position. Most importantly, find your comfortable sitting position and adjust your chair to help you maintain it.

Here are the main considerations for a healthy workspace

- Sit or stand with your shoulders centred over your hips and your spine in a neutral position. If you are sitting, start by slumping slightly, then roll your pelvis forward until you can feel yourself sitting on your 'sit' bones. Centre your shoulders over your hips and lengthen slightly from the back of your neck. Keep your feet flat on the floor
- If you have an adjustable chair, make sure you set yourself up and then the chair to support you in that position
- If you are standing, try to take weight evenly and centre your shoulders over your hips
- Your desk should be at a height so that your elbows are at 90 degrees and your wrists flat on your keyboard
- The top of your screen should be at eye height and around arm's length away. Ideally, have a screen separate from your keyboard
- Make sure you have adequate lighting
- Use headphones for taking phone calls
- Take breaks!!

112   Trish Formby

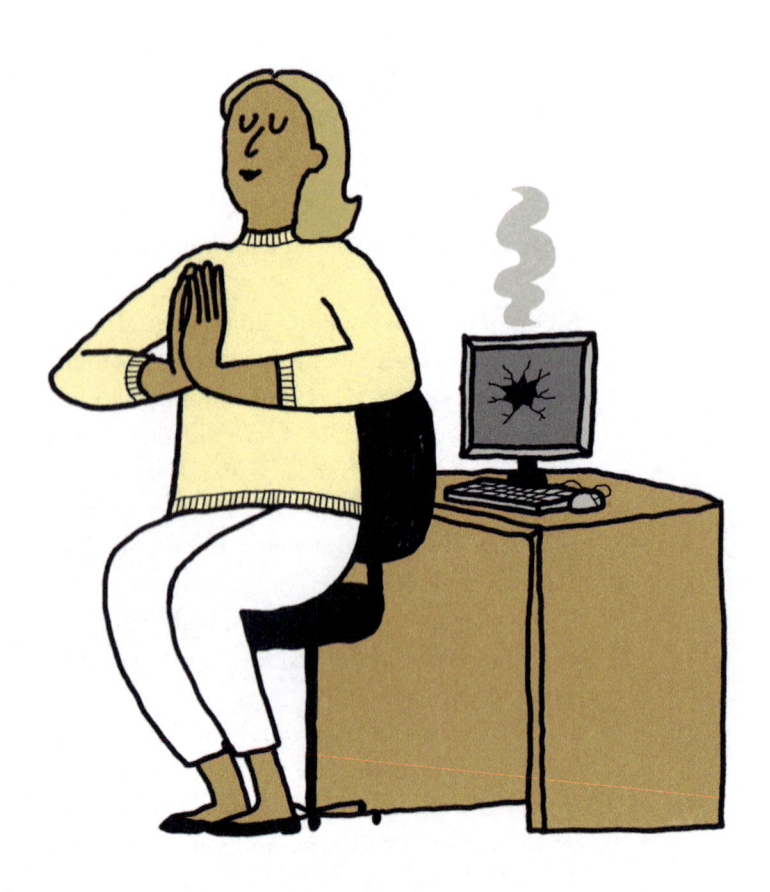

Say a Little Prayer (Wrists, Forearms)

Many of the activities we carry out during the day involve repetitive or prolonged positions of the wrist and forearms that overload the muscles causing pain and discomfort or, worse, damage to the muscles and tendons. Common instances come from work over long periods that involve gripping, operating machinery and typing.

This little exercise could not be easier, and it will be all the more beneficial in the long term if you can carry it out fairly frequently. Place your hands in the prayer position and raise your elbows up so they are level with your wrists. Feel that lovely stretch on the underside of your wrists. Hold this position for 30 seconds.

Now place the back of your hands together and lower the elbows so you feel the stretch on the top of the wrist and hold for 30 seconds.

Trish Formby

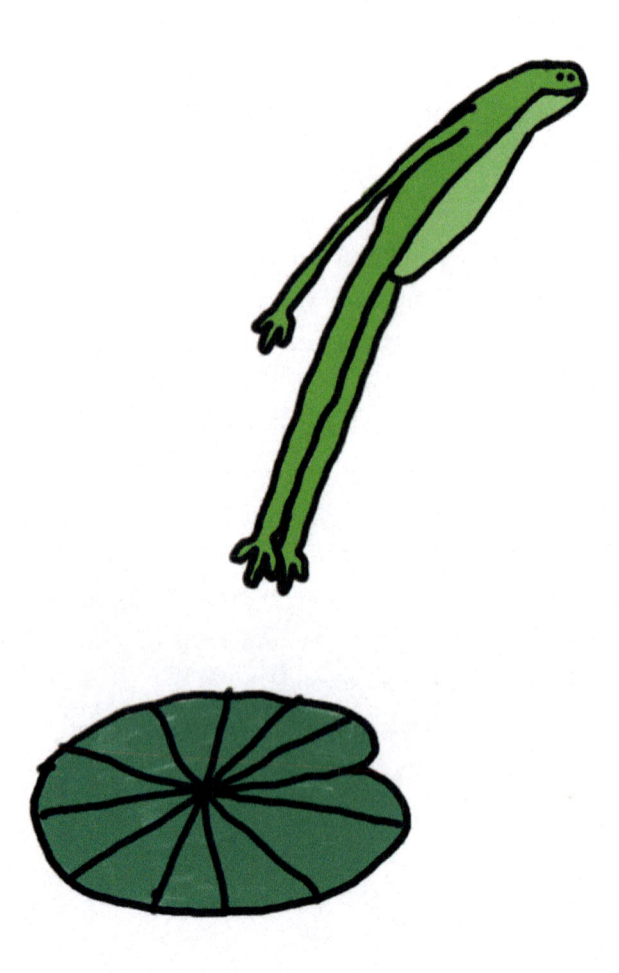

Jump To It! (Whole Body)

Hopping and jumping are things that we do all the time as children – hopscotch, skipping and jumping rope – but, as we get older, we lose our ability to bounce. Our joints and soft tissues become stiffer, we lose some balance agility and, no longer in the playground, the urge to play hopscotch or reach for the skipping rope is not quite as strong! We need to rediscover our inner child because these activities are brilliant for bone density, balance, strengthening and cardiovascular fitness.

Here's one for the adult in the home! Start by rising up and down on your toes. Try speeding up a little so you bounce back up again on the rise. Once you have got the hang of that try a few little jumps. As you grow in confidence, try hopping on one leg a few times, and then the other leg. Hold on to something for support, if you like.

It's better if you do a few at a time so that you can exploit the concept known as the 'stretch-shortening cycle'. This is when the muscles and tendons immediately shorten in response to being stretched quickly. Think of a coil spring bouncing back to its regular length after being stretched. If you start to enjoy this and feel the benefits, invest in a skipping rope – or ask your partner if they fancy a game of hopscotch or leapfrog!

116 Trish Formby

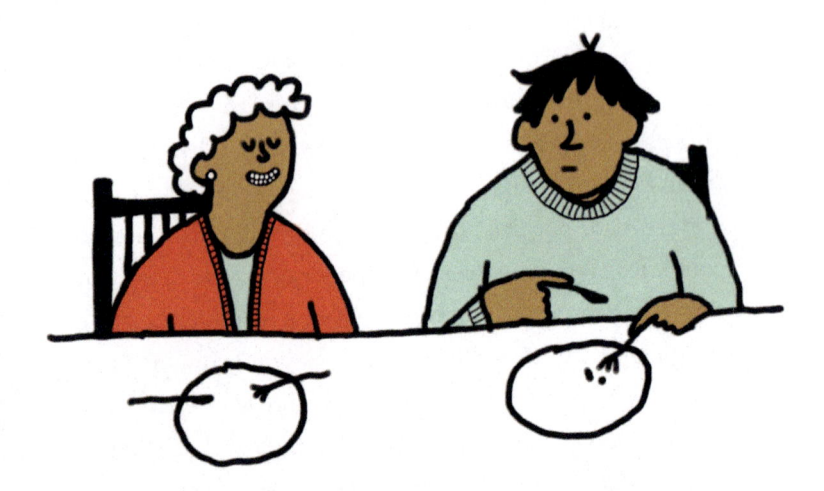

Dinner Party Diagnosis (General)

Have you ever sat down with a group of people, mentioned an ache or a pain and found that just about every person around is apparently an expert on the subject? Our friends and family love to give well-meaning advice based on their own experience or something they have read. It's the same after a quick search about your symptoms on Dr. Google. Careful – this can do more harm than good.

Just remember that there can be many differing underlying causes for pain and the symptoms that you are suffering from might sound the same as your neighbours but will probably have very different causes and require different treatment.

It's important to listen to your body and if something isn't right, go and seek a professional opinion, rather than listen to your benevolent mates and all the experts out there on the Internet.

118 Trish Formby

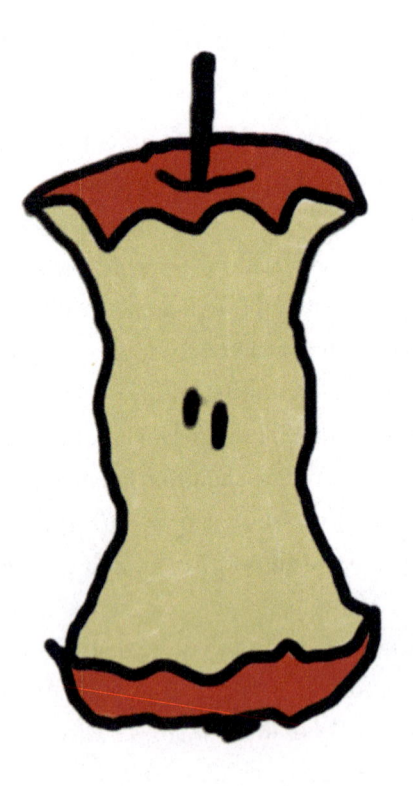

Chew On It (Jaw)

You have probably never heard of the temporomandibular joint, but you have probably just used it, and you will use it again in a few seconds. In short, this is your jaw. You can feel this joint just in front of your ear when you open and close your mouth. It can become clicky and painful in people who grind their teeth or after an injury. Stress is often a factor in teeth-grinding and jaw-clenching so general relaxation (*See* **Hit the Reset Button**) is a must. And don't chew gum, it can make jaw pain worse!

Try this exercise after you have finished brushing your teeth. Look into a mirror so you can see all your face. Place your fingertips on your chin and press your tongue to the roof of your mouth. Don't forget to lengthen at the back of the neck. Now open your mouth a few centimetres by allowing your jaw to drop downwards. Check in the mirror to see that there is no deviation of the jaw from side to side. Repeat 10 times.

Trish Formby

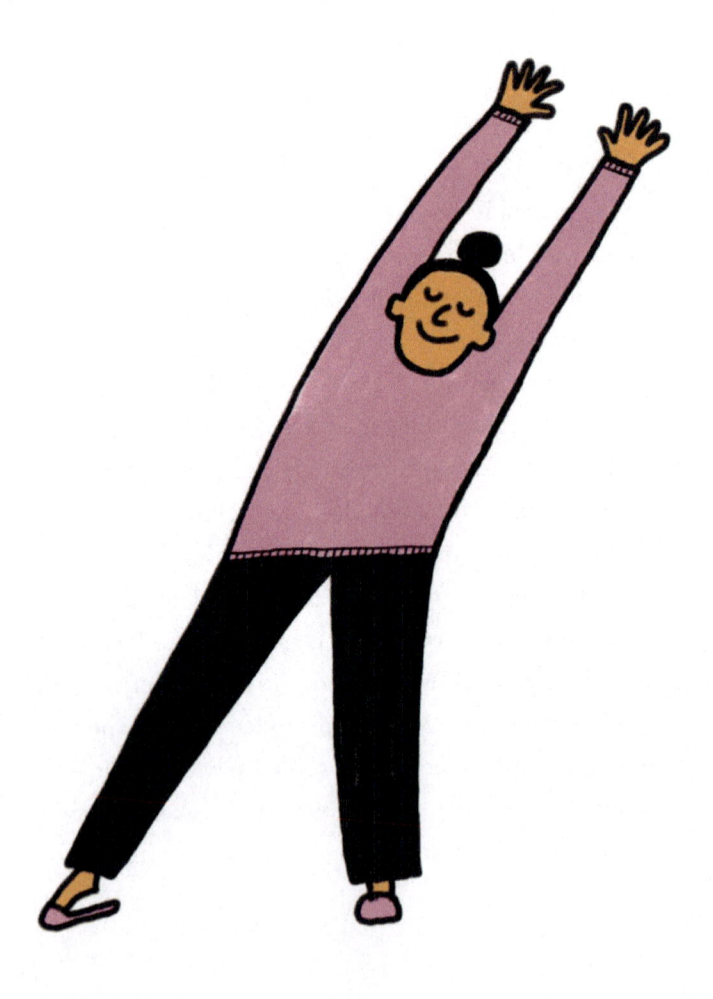

Pause for Thought and Boost the Brain (Relaxation, Mobility)

'Pause' exercises are exactly that: Taking a break and a breather during the working day to move your body, rest your brain and re-setting before continuing.

A few minutes every hour to do some simple physical exercises will help your circulation, improve oxygen flow to the brain, minimise stiffness in your joints and muscles and keep you mobile. It's also a good plan to give your mind some dedicated downtime too. Try some breathing exercises, or mindfulness, both shown to help with memory, productivity and creativity.

Set an alarm every hour until it becomes second nature. Try mixing up your breaks throughout the day so that you alternate a physical break with a mental one. You will find all the activity options right here in this book.

Trish Formby

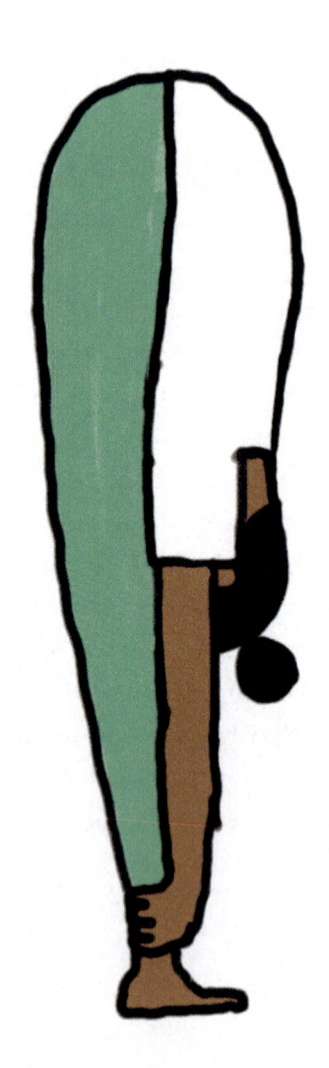

A Note on Stretching (Whole Body)

There are many different ways to stretch, and it can help to understand why and when we need to stretch – and when it is not a good idea.

We all need different levels of mobility in our joints depending on the things that we do. For instance, a gymnast will require way more flexibility in their joints than someone who enjoys hiking. The most important thing is to match our flexibility to the tasks, sports and activities that we perform regularly.

It is also really important that we have the muscle capacity to match our flexibility. Ideally, we want to maintain joint mobility with active stretches where the muscles are doing the work. The calf-raise on the stairs (**See All Rise**) is a good example where we are controlling the movement through full range AND stretching the muscle as it lengthens under load, rather than passively, where an external force pushes you into a position (e.g. another person pushing you into a stretch). You might need to use passive stretches initially to get you going, say, after an injury where there is stiffness of a joint from scar tissue or after immobilisation or tightness of a capsule (the connective tissue around our joints).

A word of warning: There are instances where stretching might be detrimental. Muscles that feel tight are not necessarily shortened. Sometimes our muscles can feel like that because they are fatigued and other times because they are trying to protect us, for instance in some cases of neural pain. In these scenarios, passive and prolonged stretching will not be the answer; active mobilisation and strengthening through range and within pain will be more beneficial.

Studies have shown that prolonged stretching of the hamstrings prior to exercise will reduce their ability to perform. That means that vigorous 'static stretching' just before running (not jogging) isn't going to enhance your performance. It may even harm. A better solution is to wake them up with some bridging exercises or try the **Horsing Around** exercise.

Another example is calves. Many recreational runners experience tightness in the calf muscles. You often see people stopping to stretch their calves out. If you're feeling brave, tell them they would be better off doing the 'eccentric' exercises to improve the endurance of their calves but perhaps don't stop to see their reaction.

Add Your Own Exercises

Add Your Own Exercises

Add Your Own Exercises

Add Your Own Exercises

Acknowledgements

This book would not have been possible without Niall Edworthy, who encouraged me to get off my butt and write it. The magnificent illustrations are by Mudd Bexley.

I would also like to thank my amazing family, especially my sisters and my husband, who all took the time to try out every one of the exercises … whilst we were meant to be on holiday together!

About Trish Formby

Trish began teaching exercise classes in the late 80s complete with Lycra, Reebok High Tops and big hair. She completed her undergraduate training as a physio in 1992 in Australia and later a Sports Master's degree before moving permanently to the UK where one thing led to another, and she never quite made it home.

Trish worked in private practice in London for many years, most of them in her clinic in Kensington where she was privileged to work with elite and professional athletes including tennis, rugby and football players, and swimmers, as well as actors, musicians and writers. It was a very vibrant and exciting time to be a physio with many new concepts in evidence-based treatment coming to the fore.

Trish was one of the first physiotherapists in London to integrate Clinical Pilates alongside manual therapy in the late nineties. Through her interest in biomechanics, she was able to combine therapies to tailor treatments for her clients in unique ways. She was also a lecturer on the sports physiotherapy course at UCL and ran her own courses on spinal rehabilitation called Integrated Rehabilitation for the Spine in the early 2000s.

Today she lives in West Sussex with her husband, two boys and her dog Banjo. Thirty years on, Trish still loves treating her patients and especially loves rehabilitation and exercise prescription. She tries most injuries out on herself. She is her own guinea pig and she still loves Lycra.

Printed in Dunstable, United Kingdom